D0189061

A PLUME BOOK

THE BLACK BOOK OF HOLLYWOOD PREGNANCY SECRETS

KYM DOUGLAS is one of the most sought-after beauty and life-style contributors on television. She began her career as a TV news journalist in Michigan. You can see her regularly on *The Ellen DeGeneres Show*, E! Television, and on the Fox number-one-rated Los Angeles morning show *Good Day LA*. Kym is the host of the nationally syndicated radio show with Jim Brickman called *Your Weekend* and has also made appearances on *Soap Talk*, *Good Day Live*, and *BEFORE & AFTERnoon*. Kym has been married to Jerry Douglas of *The Young and the Restless* for more than twenty years. They have one son and live in Los Angeles. Kym blogs and has a weekly beauty and lifestyle newsletter on her Web site, kymdouglas.com.

CINDY PEARLMAN is a leading celebrity columnist and an author of many books, including two teen novels and the film book *You Gotta See This*. She has coauthored books with Olivia Newton-John, Janice Dickinson, Carnie Wilson, Jim Brickman, and Flex Wheeler, and cowrote the bestselling *It's Not About the Horse* with Wyatt Webb and the upcoming *Jigsaw* with horse racing jockey Sylvia Harris. She is also a nationally syndicated writer for the New York Times syndicate and the *Chicago Sun-Times*. Her work has appeared in *Entertainment Weekly*, *People*, *Us Weekly*, *Good Housekeeping*, and *TV Guide*. Cindy blogs and has a celebrity and beauty newsletter on her Web site: cindypearlman.com.

Tips from . . .

Halle Berry
Milla Jovovich
Michelle Pfeiffer
Kate Hudson
Mira Sorvino
Julia Roberts
Tina Fey
Sarah Jessica Parker
Brooke Shields
Elisabeth Hasselbeck
Bobbi Brown
Helena Bonham Carter
Tori Spelling
Jenny McCarthy
Angela Bassett
Salma Hayek
Kate Beckinsale
Katie Holmes
Susan Sarandon
Gabrielle Reece
Cindy Crawford
Angie Harmon
Helen Hunt
Diane Keaton

And more . . .

The Black Book of
Hollywood
Pregnancy
Secrets

Kym Douglas
and Cindy Pearlman

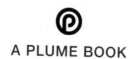

A PLUME BOOK

PLUME
Published by the Penguin Group
Penguin Group (USA) Inc., 375 Hudson Street, New York, New York 10014,
U.S.A. • Penguin Group (Canada), 90 Eglinton Avenue East, Suite 700, Toronto,
Ontario, Canada M4P 2Y3 (a division of Pearson Penguin Canada Inc.) • Penguin
Books Ltd., 80 Strand, London WC2R 0RL, England • Penguin Ireland, 25 St.
Stephen's Green, Dublin 2, Ireland (a division of Penguin Books Ltd.) • Penguin
Group (Australia), 250 Camberwell Road, Camberwell, Victoria 3124, Australia
(a division of Pearson Australia Group Pty. Ltd.) • Penguin Books India Pvt. Ltd.,
11 Community Centre, Panchsheel Park, New Delhi – 110 017, India • Penguin
Group (NZ), 67 Apollo Drive, Rosedale, North Shore 0632, New Zealand (a divi-
sion of Pearson New Zealand Ltd.) • Penguin Books (South Africa) (Pty.) Ltd., 24
Sturdee Avenue, Rosebank, Johannesburg 2196, South Africa

Penguin Books Ltd., Registered Offices: 80 Strand, London WC2R 0RL, England

First published by Plume, a member of Penguin Group (USA) Inc.

First Printing, April 2009
10 9 8 7 6 5 4 3 2 1

Copyright © Kym Douglas and Cindy Pearlman, 2009

Ⓟ REGISTERED TRADEMARK—MARCA REGISTRADA

LIBRARY OF CONGRESS CATALOGING-IN-PUBLICATION DATA

Douglas, Kym.
  The black book of Hollywood pregnancy secrets / Kym Douglas and Cindy
Pearlman.
      p. cm.
  ISBN 978-0-452-29015-0
  1. Pregnancy—California—Los Angeles. 2. Beauty, Personal. 3. Celebrities—
Health and hygiene—California—Los Angeles. 4. Motherhood—California—
Los Angeles. I. Pearlman, Cindy, 1964– II. Title.
  RG551.D68 2009
  618.2—dc22

                                                       2008051023

Printed in the United States of America
Set in Esprit Book

BOOKS ARE AVAILABLE AT QUANTITY DISCOUNTS WHEN USED TO PROMOTE PRODUCTS OR
SERVICES. FOR INFORMATION PLEASE WRITE TO PREMIUM MARKETING DIVISION, PENGUIN
GROUP (USA) INC., 375 HUDSON STREET, NEW YORK, NEW YORK 10014.

*Kym would like to dedicate this book to
the best "gift" of her life: Hunter William Douglas,
with love from your mother.*

*Cindy would like to dedicate this book to
her mom, Renee Pearlman, who is missed every single day.
And to her wonderful aunt Cheryl Davis Pearlman.
You're an amazing mom to all of us.*

*Kym and Cindy would also like to dedicate this book to
our wonderful editor and new mommy Cherise.
We hope this is your first baby book!
All our love and best wishes.*

At the hospital, I was surprised when they just let us take the baby. I was like, "You don't test us or anything?"
—**Leah Remini**

Every day is a new adventure for me. Wait. For us.
—**Christina Aguilera**

A mother's arms are more comforting than anyone else's.
—**Princess Diana**

CONTENTS

Baby, Love

Cheerleaders and Angelina Jolie. It's all their faults.

It's not enough that we had to deal with those cheerleaders in high school like we told you about in previous books, but now we have Angelina Jolie, who is the mother of the international multicultural House of Pitt. She not only parents little Shiloh, Zahara, Maddox, Pax, and the twins but also bounces back from pregnancies, has six children in tow, stars in action movies hanging her bod out of moving vehicles, and even works for the UN in her spare time.

Mother of six and spare time. We can barely type those words without breaking into hives.

What upsets us the most is that in her ninth month of pregnancy with twins, Angie looks effortlessly chic while in a black T-shirt and skinny jeans and romping on the all-so-romantic beaches of France with Brad and the brood. We ask: Is it even legal to wear skinny jeans when you're nine months pregnant with twins! Stop the madness right now!

Don't even get us started on the fact that about thirty seconds after she had that precious little Shiloh with the adorable upper lip, she's starring in a photo spread for St. John looking even thinner than she did before giving birth. We might be hallucinating, but wasn't she wearing a gold body-hugging dress in those ads just months after *push, push, shove, shove, you can do it.* Again, we would like to ask the court of women everywhere: Is this legal to make the rest of us feel so badly?

This brings us to *The Black Book of Hollywood Pregnancy Secrets.* We told you how to stay beautiful and how to stay fit in other tomes, and you said that you wanted more. The minute we decided to put pen to paper and write this book, suddenly all of Hollywood threw their birth pill controls down the toilet at the Ivy and became pregnant. We would like to apologize to the Ivy right now in the event they had any plumbing problems. But seriously, we've noticed an actual pregnancy epidemic in the 90210 area code.

So like your good beauty spies that we are, there was only one choice: We had to descend on these pregnant A-listers in movies, TV, and the music industry and find out how they (like that Angelina) could defy all the common misconceptions about being pregnant: They didn't get fat; they didn't get bloated; their ankles didn't swell that much; they didn't wear their grandmother's old clothing. Look at Nicole Richie, Gwen Stefani, and even J.Lo. All of these ladies went beyond the typical pregnancy glow and actually looked healthier and better than ever as they went into trimester three.

We wanted to know how they did it—their tips, their tricks, and their tried and true methods. Secret number one: We learned that these girls even figured out how to maneuver Mother Nature, and she's a pretty big A-lister who might even be represented by CAA and PMK, but they don't reveal client lists. But we digress.

We learned that pregnant Hollywood doesn't get fat and moody, and sit around eating bonbons or having sexy thoughts about Ben or Jerry. These full, lush, expecting women didn't lose their sex appeal but were sexier than ever.

Again, we wanted to know how they did it, so we asked them, and as always couldn't believe it when they just told us.

It wasn't enough, so we also went to their birthing coaches, their ob-gyns, their pregnancy masseuses, their Lamaze class teachers, their yoga instructors, their nannies-to-be, their nursery designers, their organic baby food makers, and their makeup artists, skin care experts, and personal trainers. The point was to find out what made these ultra-hot mamas able to go through the same nine months all the rest of us have to go through, but in great style and spirit—and without stretch marks.

Stars don't have the luxury that many of us do after giving birth. They're expected to get right back out there looking thinner and more gorgeous than ever. Paparazzi surround them the minute they give birth, and the pressure is on before they even leave the hospital steps and step into the Beemer.

We wondered how they coped with common pregnancy beauty problems including acne, pregnancy mask, thinning hair, hair dye vs. no hair dye, and feeling big as a house while not feeling sexy. How did the stars pump up their own self-esteem and remain desirable for their mates? How did they handle the idea of not using certain products anymore—and what advice did they follow? How did they cope with the weight gain and cravings? How do you breast-feed and feed the media?

The Black Book of Hollywood Pregnancy Secrets jumps right into Hollywood's current baby boom and the mass media's obsession with stars who have baby bumps and little ones in those ultra-cool strollers that cost more than some small condos.

We love Halle Berry for telling us there isn't a potato chip in the land that she could resist while pregnant. Former model Milla Jovovich said that several bagels with peanut butter was her breakfast for nine months. We won't mention how a certain supermodel managed to pop out three children and pop into a diamond-encrusted Victoria's Secret bra and walk the runway in what seemed like two days. How! Why!

How do the stars exercise, and what are their secrets for getting in shape so much faster than the rest of us? And what do they do to lose the weight after baby is born? What is the beauty regime of busy mom of twins Angela Bassett that takes only five minutes? How does Kate Hudson cope with a sullen toddler and still manage to look fab and go out on dates? How did Mira Sorvino drop more than eighty pounds after being pregnant for eighteen months over three years with her two children? Mira, we bow to you.

Kym, who is the mother of ten-year-old Hunter Douglas, remembers being pregnant this way: "I remember, Cindy, being so bloated that my height was almost equal to my circumference. I was as wide as I was tall. I'm only five feet tall. My belly button hurt because it stuck out so much. I couldn't sleep because I couldn't get comfortable. I had swollen feet and ankles. I had so much water retention that I literally would swoosh when I walked. All of my clothes looked like granny wear. Don't get me started about those extra-large bras and those huge undies." P.S.: Hunter, if you ever read this, Mommy loves you, but when you grow up you should remember this paragraph. And please clean your room more because look what I went through to have you!

Cindy is sitting here reading Kym's words feeling very, very nervous. Yes, it's true that she has those same granny pants, but it was only for regular weight gain during her short tenure on the Chicago Fox Network. But then, of course, Cindy and Kym wrote *The Black Book of Hollywood Diet Secrets* and the granny pants were burned just like Tori did on that great episode of *Tori & Dean: Inn Love*. We love you, Tori, and naturally Ms. Spelling was nice enough to give us some secrets later in the book. Congrats on baby Stella.

Tori was not alone. You want stars with bellies ready to pop? We talked to Gwyneth, Liv, Jessica, Halle, Kate and Katie (Mrs. Tommy Cruise), Nicole, Gwen, Christina, Madonna, and our favorite earth mother, Susan Sarandon. And we couldn't resist asking a few of the impending famed fathers for their helpful hints, which include Matthew McConaughey on diapering and Jack Black on teaching your son to be a rock star.

We've got our very own Five-Minute Mom Makeover, hot beauty tips for pregnancy, and many heartwarming A-list stories about stars and their offspring. We even had to sneak around and present our typical blind items, which now we're calling *Overheard in a Beverly Hills Delivery Room*. Plus we have the latest and greatest products of all sorts, from beauty to baby booty, that will help any new mom feel glam while taking on the greatest role of her life.

In the end, we even had this pregnant pause.

Kym was trying to counsel Cindy on motherhood and offered these words of wisdom: "Through it all, no matter what stories you hear and whatever you see, having a child is the greatest gift and the greatest blessing you can ever have in your life. It fills you with more joy than you'll ever know. And always remember one important thing—your stomach will never be the same, so you'll have to suck it in for the rest of your life and Spanx will become your best friend."

"But Kym," Cindy said, "Spanx are already my best friend, and I only have a dog."

Overheard in a Beverly Hills Delivery Room: This starlet is so demanding that despite giving birth at the horrid hour of three in the morning, which is when the little Hollywood tyke decided to make his debut, she still insisted that her hair stylist, makeup artist, and celebrity newborn photographer immediately meet her in her swanky birthing suite at Cedars-Sinai. Miss Movie Star insisted that she needed a straight blow-dry after giving birth because her hair had frizzed during her C-section. She was also concerned about her face, so her makeup artist gave her the full job because God forbid she looked tired in that heinous fluorescent lighting that Cedars and all hospitals stubbornly insist on. (We can see her point of view on that one—fluorescent lighting is very harsh! So we can't blame her—just kidding.) When the nurse came in with her newborn bundle of joy, she had to put breast-feeding for the first time on hold because she was in the middle of a close-up for photos she planned to FedEx out the next day to *People* and *Us Weekly*.

CHAPTER 1

Yummy Mommies

I love being pregnant. You feel more like a woman than you've ever felt before. You just feel like everything about your body is there for your baby. It feels great.

—**Angelina Jolie**

A-LIST MOMMY: THE GREAT KATE

Kate Hudson doesn't just have a sunny attitude but believes in a positive, sunny way of life. Alas, she says that as a mom (to three-year-old Ryder), you can't always be the poster mom for shiny, happy parenthood. "You do say the worst things, like because I said so," says a horrified Kate.

"I say it all the time," Hudson says with a giggle. She adds, "One morning I got so exasperated because Ryder was so grumpy. He was making me into a grump. Well, that morning he didn't like anything I made for breakfast. I just got so mad that I said, 'We are happy people! Do you understand! We are happy people!' It was the only thing I could come up with."

Hudson says her life has changed since her divorce from rocker husband Chris Robinson.

"I do find it tough to date," she admits. "It's just different now. I'd rather be home with my son cooking dinner than going out with a guy. My son is my man. I love waking up in the morning and having Ryder come in shouting, 'Mommy get up.' I'm just the happiest ever.

"I do want to meet someone who really understands my priorities, which is my child. Maybe I'll meet someone with children. That's what happened to my mom and dad. Both had children," she says. "It will take a special man who loves both me and Ryder.

"I don't even feel like a single mom," she says. "My ex-husband is still around so much that I don't feel like I'm single in the best way. It's been a surprising and wonderful time because this divorce was something both Chris and I wanted. We both still love each other. I can't believe I got so lucky."

BB EXPERTS: ELLIE MILLER AND MELISSA GOULD OF THE BABY PLANNERS

"We take the labor out of your delivery," promises Ellie Miller and Melissa Gould. Their hot new company is called the Baby Planners, and they make being a new mommy—celebrity or civilian—a much easier task.

Ellie is a former network news producer and manager for various news organizations including CNN and Channel One. Melissa is an award-winning television writer/producer whose work has appeared everywhere from NBC to the Disney Channel. Aside from the births of their own children, Ellie's and Melissa's professional and personal experiences have lead to their greatest production to date: The Baby Planners.

"We were born in the fall of 2006 but didn't come out to the public until spring 2007. We spent about nine months researching the industry, which seems appropriate," Melissa says.

What do the Baby Planners do for both their A-list clients and mere mortals?

"We try to fulfill all of our clients' needs with half-hour phone consultations. We can spend a half hour on one topic. You'd be surprised by how much we can cover in thirty minutes. A lot of parents are excited. They're hormonal. We're here to help," Ellie says.

Specifically, the ladies will answer anything and everything. You want advice on nipple cream? They'll tell you which is their favorite. You want to know about the latest in organic diapers? They're available to go green with you. They even do registry consultation to figure out tastes, style, trends, and budgets. "We also stock the nursery. There is nothing we haven't been able to fulfill yet," Melissa says.

The Black Book had to ask: What is the wildest request they've ever received? "The weirdest call was when I was asked what time of year was the best time to have a baby and if I could provide a name—which we don't do," Ellie says, laughing.

"Even when working with celebs, it's the same questions. All parents want the same thing—a little reassurance, a little help navigating through the products. We try to be the voice of reason, and we're not a mother-in-law or best friend. We're neutral," Melissa says.

The Baby Planners don't talk about their A-list names, but they say that both famed mommies and daddies have called. "We love it when we talk to the husbands as much as the wives," Ellie says. "The husbands usually get involved when buying technical equipment like the strollers. We also go out on shopping excursions with the moms, the grandmother, the sisters, and the friends."

The Baby Planners can cut through all the choice vs. not-so-hot products out there, too.

"There is so much stuff," Ellie says. "The trend is toward organic, and it's all overwhelming. Parents want to do the right thing, and we stay on top of it for them. We stay on the trends. We mom-test and kid-test the products. Sometimes it's the kids who will give you the very best reviews."

"Or the worst," says Melissa.

BB: Okay, you've just found out that you're pregnant. What are the first few things a new mommy should think about doing?

Melissa: The first thing you should do is take care of yourself. There aren't really many things you need to take home a baby.

Ellie: Your body is changing. Listen to your body. That's your major job right now. If you're tired during a new part of the day, then take a moment. If you're starving, you need to eat. Don't deprive yourself of what your body is telling you that you need.

Melissa: Also, people are excited and want to help you. Don't feel you can do it all on your own. Let your friends pick up your groceries for you. People need a task, and let them help you. That goes for adoptive couples and surrogates. The same rules apply. Having a baby is an emotionally driven time no matter how you're having it. Listen to your body and let your friends and family help you now.

BB: You've said that any mom needs only five things to take a baby home. What's on that list?

Melissa: First you need a car seat; we're big on getting a car seat professionally installed. Some 80 percent of infant car seats are installed in the wrong way. A lot times it's very reasonable or free to have that seat installed. It's really important.

Ellie: There's a lot of stress in choosing a stroller. That's one of the five things. We love those Graco Snug-Rides, a stroller frame that the infant car seat snaps right into. It's great if you're not ready to splurge on the Bugaboo or you don't want to figure it out. It's the same thing with the high chair. You don't need one until about six months old. Don't give in to that added pressure right after giving birth. Just get what you need. Your baby needs a place to sleep—either a crib or a bassinet. People stress over cribs. You don't need a crib right away. Your baby won't be in it.

Melissa: If it's not there in the nursery, it's okay. Most nurseries are not perfect right away.

BB: Even if you're Nicole Kidman's new child, you really don't need a complete wardrobe yet . . . do you?

Melissa: You need the basic onesies. We recommend swaddling blankets—they are fabulous and will help you in the first few weeks. By the way, wash everything you get at your shower before the baby is born.

Ellie: Melissa loves the Bouncer Chair, which she calls Mommy's first shower. It's a simple chair that vibrates so you have a moment for yourself. Some babies love swings, but they're not for everybody.

We're also big fans of diapers.com. You can do so much online—it's a great thing to get someone a gift certificate from this place. You can do anything from organic diapers to flushable diapers.

BB: How organic do you think you need to be these days?

Melissa: It depends on the person. If you're interested in putting a toe into organics, try cloth diapers when you're at home. When you're out you can do your Huggies. You don't have to do it all at once.

Ellie: If you're already living a green lifestyle, it will be a smooth transition. If not, split the difference: green at home, but if you're out and need to change and feed your baby, then do the other stuff. If it's not for you, then forget about it.

BB: Where do you stand on breast-feeding?

Melissa: By all means, try it. You don't have to commit for two years. Some women have a lot of difficulty with it and beat themselves up. We have a lot of fabulous lactation experts who can come into your home. After that, if it's still not working for you, then your mental health takes over and some great bottles take over.

BB: What do moms always forget to buy before giving birth?

Melissa: The feminine things that you need, like nipple cream.

Ellie: After you give birth you're really sore. We have clients put a maxi pad in the freezer. It's very soothing, although hard to wrap your head around it. We put it in our nursery necessity package. We always have extra diapers and wipes ready for new moms. People don't buy enough, but they're nervous to run out of the house. Overstocking isn't a bad thing.

Melissa: We have a necessity package including diapers, wipes, Q-tips, cotton balls, different things for cradle cap, some balms for diaper rash. We also put in belly butter for mom for stretch marks. And we include a swaddling blanket.

BB: Any product you've found to be a real lifesaver?

Melissa: A lot of our clients are anti-pacifier. We say to have
           one just in case. A lot of them are organics.

Ellie: There are so many great slings and carriers, and our
           clients are really comfortable in them. It's hands-free
           baby wearing and a great way for baby to bond with
           mommy or daddy. The baby is so snuggly inside that
           sling. In fact, it makes them feel like they're back in
           the womb.

BB: Are women trying too hard to look like the Holly-
           wood women five seconds after giving birth? What
           else do they beat themselves up about?

Melissa: There is a lot of pressure everywhere. We want our
           clients to give themselves a break. Women do want
           to get back into shape and they see these actresses
           immediately back into their size 4 jeans.

Ellie: Here in LA, baby is in utero and the moms are con-
           cerned about preschool placement. That industry is
           booming, and it starts before your baby is born. We
           had one client with whom we talked about that more
           than anything.

Melissa: Our whole thing is don't judge. We felt under pres-
           sure to do it all when we had our children. Our mo-
           tivation is to make it easier and ask for help if you're
           feeling stressed and unnerved before the arrival of
           your baby or overwhelmed after the baby is here.
           We're here to hold hands.

Overheard in a Beverly Hills Delivery Room: "There
comes a time in pregnancy when there is just no sucking it in

anymore. I went right for the big fluffy robes at the end." —Julia Roberts on her weight gain with her twins, Hazel and Finn, and new baby, Henry.

UBER A-LIST MOTHER: ANGELINA JOLIE

Yes, we were joking earlier about the uber mother of our time, Angelina Jolie. We bow to the mother of six who also acts and has a guy in her life named Brad Pitt. On a cold winter morning, the Black Book caught up with Angelina at the Regency Hotel in New York City. Looking beyond gorgeous and teeny-tiny in a red sweater and black pants, the effortlessly chic and friendly Jolie provided a few mom secrets for us. Thanks, Angie!

BB: How do you juggle everything?

AJ: I plan a lot obsessively. I'm very, very lucky I love the different elements of my life—I love being with my kids, I love being with Brad. There is just nothing that's better. This is the life I chose to have.

BB: What do Brad and the children bring to your life?

AJ: A lot of fun. They're just a joy. Brad and the children bring a joy of life that exists nowhere else.

BB: Will you work with Brad?

AJ (laughing): Who will watch the children?

BB: How do you make things fun for your family when the paparazzi are basically stalking you?

AJ: I've made a point not to let it change my life other than I carefully plan my holidays, where we go and where we stay, to ensure some quality of life that's private and nice for the kids. Otherwise we simply don't let it affect us. The only time it's hard is when the kids want to go somewhere. I've had so many people offer to take my kids to Disneyland or trick or treating for me. I don't want to ever do that. I want to take them ourselves. We find ways to do it as a family. There are worse problems to have than rumors.

BB: You went trick or treating last year?

AJ: We were in India and Brad, the kids, and I had an odd celebration in the hotel where we were staying. We had candy sent up, which we said was from the saints. Z had an afro on her. I had dreadlocks.

BB: What defines a good personal relationship to you?

AJ: I think you have to be honest. I don't want to spend my life pretending to be someone else. I don't ever want the person next to me to pretend. We have a long life ahead of us. You have to be who you are. It's the only way you will be truly happy.

BB: How do you juggle work and the kids?

AJ: The thing that helps make the decision is how long it is shooting. I haven't shot more than seven weeks on a movie in two years. I need to spend time with my kids.

A-LIST MOMMY: HAVE A GOOD FEY

"I don't care how many covers you're on when you're chasing a three-year-old around with a pull up hoping she won't poop on the floor. You're just like every other mom on the planet," says America's favorite funny woman, Tina Fey, who starred in *Baby Mama*.

Yes, she has been called a comic geek goddess who is leading a laugh revolution, but she's also mom to a three-year-old. Fey could riff forever on motherhood. She and husband, Jeff Richmond, are the proud parents of Alice, who was born in September 2005.

"My daughter likes to watch people get their makeup done. When I come home she goes, 'You got makeup? I like your makeup? Who did your eyes?' I have a very girly girl on my hands.

"She also likes the snack table, but who doesn't?" Fey says with a laugh.

Fey says juggling movies, TV, and motherhood requires more than she has at times.

"I'm very, very ill. I'm not doing well," she jokes. "No, the truth is I work and then whatever other time I have I'm with my daughter. And then I go to sleep.

"I think that you basically have to abandon the dreams of having any other adult activities in your life," she says. "You just have to go to sleep whenever your child goes to sleep. That's basically how we're doing it."

She says the 2008 writers' strike gave her some R&R.

"I stayed home with my daughter," she says. "That was sort of the only blessing of the strike. It was a little bit like a maternity leave that I didn't have when my daughter was born.

"I also did my union duty on the picket line," she says.

Fey says that she likes to bring her daughter to work. "I do try to bring her sometimes, and she likes to come. She likes to hang out in the makeup room.

"It always brightens my day to have my daughter around," she says.

"Now I'm back at work and it's tough because my daughter is old enough to say, 'No, you not go to work! You not go outside,'" she says.

With a sigh she adds, "It's hard for any working parents."

HELLO ON HIGH HEELS

Recently rated the most comfortable heel by the *Wall Street Journal*, it's no wonder celebs have taken a liking to the new four-inch heel by Taryn Rose International. Spotted recently on a very pregnant Angelina Jolie, the new Calexa peep toe is proof that you can wear the highest of heels yet still be comfortable. Originally created by an orthopedic surgeon to give the fashion industry a high-fashion shoe with high comfort, the heels weren't intended to be made above two inches.

Now, in its tenth year of giving men and women an alternative to painful footwear, Taryn Rose has graduated to making a comfortable, elegant four-inch heel. If a six-month pregnant glamazon like Angelina Jolie is wearing them, imagine what they will feel like for the rest of us. Eight-month-pregnant-with-twins Jolie wore the heels to the *Changeling* photocall at the Palais des Festivals during the 61st Cannes International Film Festival.

Hollywood Speak: Bro-mance—When you're pregnant and your husband hangs out with his best male friend from time to time just to get away from all the female stuff like cravings and morning sickness and size 16 undies. You say, "Yes,

Brad is hanging out with George again tonight for some guy time. I think they're doing dinner and a movie. They're having a bro-mance!"

A-LIST MOMMY: SARAH JESSICA PARKER

Forget nights with Mr. Big. It's all about the little guy for her. Our favorite style queen Sarah Jessica Parker says that she likes nights at home with little James and husband Matthew Broderick.

"Honestly, we'll play blocks with him—he's really, really, really into Lego right now. He's really into *Star Wars*, and he's very into Barack Obama, on his own. He's really into this election. Really truly, he's into this election. He's come to this conclusion on his own, based specifically on Barack's gender. He's that deep. Anyway, I would do anything. Honestly, we'd basically do anything with him. Brushing his teeth is enjoyable. Right at the time when we are putting him to bed we do the teeth, and it's great."

As for her parenting tips, SJP tells the *Black Book* that James is large now and . . . in charge! "He pretty much dictates a lot of the entertainment we see, what we are going to talk about, and what we are going to do," she says, long curls flowing over on a Saturday morning at the Regency Hotel in New York City. "That's fine with me. I pretty much love to do everything with him, as long as he'll have me around. I know it's just a matter of time before he doesn't want me around. It happens. It's a developmental stage.

"You want them to get there and seek some independence. Right now, he is pretty taken with both my husband and myself," she says with a sigh of relief.

A-LIST MOMMY: BROOKE SHIELDS

It's a jungle in there.

There is Brooke Shields's New York kitchen where phones are ringing, noodles are bubbling on the stove, and a little girl is making demands of her famous mother.

What gets between Brooke and a phone interview?

Her name is Grier Hammond, two, who interrupts Mommy's talking with a major announcement.

"My baby just pointed to her eyes and said, 'Crying! I'm crying!'" Shields says, laughing. "She wants to make it clear that I shouldn't be on the phone when she's crying.

"It's just judgment, all the time," jokes the forty-two-year-old beauty who starred on NBC's *Lipstick Jungle.*

Shields says, "Grier has been coming to the set of my series, and now she runs around the house saying, 'Ki-yet.' That translates into quiet, which is what they say on the set a lot to a young girl who doesn't like to be ki-yet."

Shields sounds like any other harried working mom, with a twist.

"Sometimes I go to a restaurant to learn my lines. Our apartment in New York is small and it's impossible to find quiet," she says.

Shields doesn't have time to dwell on herself.

"What's funny about my own life is I amaze even myself with how much I do. My girlfriends are the same," she says. "The men in our lives look at us like, 'You're nuts. How can you do everything in one day?' They really don't get how much a woman can do in one morning.

"I know if I'm not doing ten things in one day, then something is wrong. I'm having an off day," she says. "In fact, if I'm only doing five things at once it's like I'm leading a life of leisure, and I get angry. I think, 'I want to do ten things.'"

Shields says that she forces herself to relax.

"You get pockets of time," she says. "That's what is great about living in New York. You stop and grab a coffee and see your friends. You grab the time."

She says motherhood has been an amazing ride for her.

"I try to find a way to slow down every day and do something one-on-one with each child. Yes, sometimes it's overwhelming because so many different things are thrown at you at once. But I get so much from everything thrown at me.

"I even get a little greedy and think, 'You asked for it all and now you even want more,'" she laughs.

GOOD EATS, MAMA

Our friend and celebrity nutritionist Cynthia Pasquella tells stars like Elisha Cuthbert, Shannon Elizabeth, and Kate Beckinsale what to eat. We asked her for a quick list of healthy substitutes for pregnancy cravings. The idea is to satisfy your craving without putting on too much weight.

Let's look at a few interesting subs:

- Ice cream. Opt for nonfat frozen yogurt, which will meet your calcium needs without the added calories.
- Chocolate. Try nonfat chocolate syrup drizzled on top of some fresh fruit.
- Candy and sweets. Substitute dried fruits such as apricots or fresh tropical fruit such as mango or pineapple.
- Salty snacks. Opt for popcorn sprinkled with herb blends or sesame breadsticks with spicy mustard dip.
- Sour snacks. Squeeze some lemon on your fish or use in a salad instead of indulging in empty calorie or sugary lemonade.

If all else fails, Cynthia says to just throw the baby belly to the wind and indulge—sometimes you have to give in! Just remember, you're eating for two—not ten!

SWOLLEN FEET, FAT ANKLES, NO PROBLEM

In Hollywood they call it cankles (when your legs and ankles become one large stump), and you don't want to be caught dead on the red carpet with this affliction. But we know that when you're pregnant your feet can't help but get swollen easily, even if your name is Nicole or Jessica. Preggers stars get puffy down below because of poor circulation and water retention. BB to the rescue: We found this Hollywood stylist trick to solve the crankle problem:

Use hot and cold footbaths to relive the swelling—soak your feet in hot water for a few seconds (without burning yourself, please), then in cold water for thirty seconds. Hot water will bring the blood to your feet, aiding circulation, while cold water moves it out of the body.

A-LIST MOMMY: GWYNETH PALTROW

She makes it look so effortless—stardom, motherhood, married to a rock star from Coldplay, and even that cute new curly bob. Who doesn't want to be Gwyneth Paltrow—at least for a day? We asked the Oscar winner a few quick questions about how she manages motherhood to little Apple and baby Moses.

BB: You starred in the action film *Iron Man* after giving birth to your son, Moses. How do you go from pregnant to doing major movie stunts for a big summer flick? Were you already in good shape before you began?

GP: No, I wish. I was like post-baby nightmare woman. (She laughs.) Seriously, I worked really, really hard and had an amazing trainer. I worked out twice a day and even did cardio dance. I felt like a complete nerd, of course, but I just worked hard because I knew this was going to be a physically demanding role. And slowly I got into shape.

BB: What were you passionate about as a little girl that you want to share with your own kids?

GP: I was really passionate about those old musicals like *Mary Poppins* and the Haley Mills movies. I was obsessed when I was little, so I've already shown *Mary Poppins* to my kids. And I'm sure I'll be showing them many more as they get older.

BB: Does Chris (Martin) sing to the children?

GP: Oh, yes, all the time. He sings lullabies. He'll sing funny joke songs. They love his music.

BB: How do you balance having a tremendous career with personal life satisfaction?

GP: Basically, I have the luxury of saying that I've done everything that I wanted to do career-wise. I mean, at a very young age I achieved a lot. So now I have the freedom to shift my focus and fully dive into this domestic kind of bliss. It might be a different story if I hadn't achieved what I wanted to achieve.

BB: You grew up with a working mother. Did you want your mom to be home more for you?

GP: I never felt like she wasn't around. I mean, I can probably point to two memories in my childhood where I came home and I was like, "Oh, Mommy's working" and it was kind of a big deal. But mostly I always knew that I could go to her. I think that I was in third grade and she was doing a film with Martin Sheen. The house they were shooting in was about six blocks from our own house and they had somehow worked this out. So we would come home from school and walk over there. It was a fantastic thing. Also, I loved being around actors; it was such a lively kind of atmosphere, everyone was creative, and it was a lovely way to grow up. I don't look at it like, "Oh, no, I'm subjecting my kids to something that's not great," because I really feel that it will be great for them.

BB: Before Apple was born did your mom give you one good piece of advice about being a mother?

GP: She's very supportive of me. It's more of a dialogue that we still have with questions about raising children. She tells me what I was like as a child. She'll give me something to go off of. It's not like, "How do I do this?" I read about five hundred books on breast-feeding, child psychology, raising a child, sleep, all that kind of stuff.

Hollywood Speak: The Infantini—A juicy alcoholic drink served at showers and made to be consumed by everyone but the preggers guest of honor. We also love another drink called the Gin 'N Colic.

CHAPTER 2

America's Next Top Maternity Model

How to Have a Glam Pregnancy

Bringing up six children is harder than making an action movie.
—**Angelina Jolie**

Moms of teenagers know why animals eat their young.
—**Unknown**

HALLE AND THE BABY BERRY

She had the cutest baby bump. It stuck out a little bit from the black silk dress like it was the bump designed by Hollywood.

Halle Berry was so delighted with the idea of having a baby that she couldn't contain her glee. "This is the greatest thing that could ever have happened to me," says the screen beauty.

What were the good and bad parts of being pregnant? "There was no bad. No morning sickness, no vomiting, no hot sweats. None of that. I loved every second of it," Berry, forty-one, says on an early Sunday morning in New York City.

Long hair falling softly on her shoulders, she pushes her bangs out of her face and mentions there were cravings during the past four months. "Get me some potato chips or some hot spicy nachos," she said. "I know women who say it's all about the sweets and cookies. For me it's all about the salty and the spicy. Pass the taco chips!"

Berry says that beyond diet, she spent her pregnancy "getting all sorts of motherhood advice. It seems like I'd get advice all day long."

One of her most pressing concerns was how to not wear those ugly tentlike pregnancy outfits. "I feel like I've been a slave to fashion all of my life," Berry says. "I had a hard time fathoming me in those huge maternity tops. I wore normal clothes until at least the last month or so."

And if she had to wear some muumuu-like creations it's not like she'd be on any red carpets or sets.

What did she do to reduce stress? "I painted. I set up a studio. I spent time with Gabriel, friends, and family. I'm even keeping a journal about this time in my life."

And she's already thinking about expanding the brood. "I'm ready for more. My age dictates that I think about it. Two would be nice."

AND NOW A PREGNANT PAUSE: A FEW BEAUTY TIPS FOR EXPECTANT MOMS

Great tips flood Black Book HQs on a daily basis. We did a quick roundup of our favorites for those with a bambino in their future:

- There will be no champagne, no Cosmos, and no cold brews for you while pregnant, even on the red carpet after the most dreadful premiere. But that doesn't mean your hubby, costars, agent, significant other, or family members aren't going to indulge in a cold one while the expectant mother is around. We don't want you to drink alcohol, but you can get something out of the deal, including better skin. When you're pregnant your skin can become much more sensitive and irritated. That's where a nice bottle of beer can come in handy. The barley, wheat, corn, rice, and hops can help invigorate your face. Pour the cold beer onto a washcloth until damp. Place on your face and leave for thirty minutes. Remove the cloth and you'll see radiant, beer-treated skin. We'll drink to that.

Just when you thought that you might not like how gorgeous Catherine Zeta-Jones is when wearing no makeup and running around Majorca, we must stop and admire her savvy skin care secrets. The mama of two keeps her porcelain skin looking soft, subtle, and youthful with an inexpensive at-home concoction anyone can whip up. To moisturize and exfoliate her skin, CZJ says she jumps in the shower after a workout and uses a mixture of honey and sea salt on her moist skin. No word if Michael joins her.

How do you de-puff a pregnancy face? Rosewater is a proven anti-inflammatory that relieves swelling. Try C.O. Bigelow Rose Water Tonic ($24 at cobigelow.com). Just spray a little mist onto a cotton pad and then dab under your eyes or other areas of puff. You'll see results in minutes.

Want an all-natural makeup remover? We know that you're probably not going to be wearing tons of eye makeup every minute into your ninth month, but if you

do go to an event while pregnant, it helps not to use per-
fumed or chemical removers to take off the makeup once
you're back in your Beverly Hills mansion. Upcoming
moms like to stay au natural with everything, so here is a
Black Book recipe for a gentle and effective eye makeup
remover. Through trial and error, we found that castor
oil is great at removing eye makeup. Even the heaviest
stuff will glide off effortlessly with this formula:

1 tablespoon canola oil
1 tablespoon castor oil
1 tablespoon light olive oil

Mix the oils together in a small, shallow glass bowl.
Pour a small amount of oil onto a cotton pad and wipe
over your eyes to remove makeup.

We also found a great pregnancy hair conditioner that
you'll need because hormones will create havoc on your
hair. Did we mention your hair might also pull more tricks
than Julia Roberts did in *Pretty Woman*? If you have naturally curly hair, it could become bone straight. ("Please,
God, please," Cindy prays.) If you have straight hair, you
will suddenly have curls. And let's not forget how it will
instantly fall out in chunks when least expected. We don't
have a cure, but we do have a quick and easy way to condition your ever-changing hair. Bananas and honey are excellent sources of potassium and vitamins A, B, and C,
which help replenish dry, damaged hair and add shine. We
love this quick recipe: Mix together one mashed banana
and one tablespoon of honey, until you have a smooth con-
sistency. Apply to damp or wet hair, put on a shower cap,
and let sit for twenty minutes. Shampoo and condition as
usual. And get ready to SHINE!

We also know how you can get what we call Sexy Mama Curls, because when you're with child everything should be touchable and soft. Hair spray, glues, and mousse can make hair sticky and stiff—especially when using a curling iron or Velcro or electric rollers. To help yourself get this touchable, mix a few drops of leave-in conditioner into your hair gel to get the hold without the crunch.

Hollywood Speak: Epidurable—The glow a woman has just before she is going to give birth! For example: "I haven't seen Nicole in months because she's been stuck in Nashville, but now that she's nine months, she's just so epidurable."

BELLY BANDIT

We've heard of getting a wrap, but this takes it to the next level. Moms struggling with a postpartum belly in LA are buying up the Belly Bandit as a way to enjoy their prepregnancy body in a healthy way. Belly Bandits are abdominal compression wraps; they have been used therapeutically for years, and now are tailored to a new mom's body after giving birth. They are designed to bring the body back to its prepregnancy form faster than ever.

"What a genius idea. This is a great gift for all new moms," says Poppy Montgomery of the popular CBS series *Without a Trace*. She and Adam Kaufman became the parents of Jackson Phillip Devereaux Kaufman on December 23, 2007, in Los Angeles.

"I love it! I'm going to have my next dance partner on the show wear it so it will keep him up straight and not slouching. I want to wear one, too—this is great!" says Karina Smirnoff of *Dancing with the Stars*.

How does it work? The Belly Bandit is an abdominal compression wrap designed to help reduce the swelling of the uterus, decrease bloating caused by water retention, support the legs and back, and provide additional support for breast-feeding moms. The increased and constant pressure it provides against the abdominal area has numerous benefits—including flattening the belly and redefining the waistline while helping to keep the back straight, which minimizes associated pain and fatigue. Breathable and comfortable to wear under all clothing with a seamless and inconspicuous fit, the Belly Bandit wrap gives new moms the support and confidence they deserve after childbirth.

Dr. Jay Goldberg, a Beverly Hills ob-gyn, says, "I recommend the Belly Bandit to any patient in the postpartum period, whether recovering from a vaginal delivery or a C-section. The Belly Bandit abdominal wrap encourages better posture, abdominal support, and self-confidence."

If you have your doctor's approval, the Belly Bandit can be worn snuggly around the waist as soon as the day after the baby is born—even after a C-section. In fact, wearing it after a C-section may actually decrease the post-op recovery time by minimizing associated incision pain, which allows greater mobility post-surgery. For maximum benefits, it should be worn day and night (removed only to shower) for six to eight weeks post-delivery. It should fit snugly with constant pressure on the belly but without any impact on breathing or circulation or discomfort to the ribs.

The Belly Bandit Collection can be purchased online at belly bandit.com and soon at local retailers for the suggested prices of $39.95 (Original), $49.95 (Couture), and $59.95 (Bamboo).

STRIKING OIL

Somehow during all the reporting on the oil crisis, we've failed to see Anderson Cooper report this on CNN: Due to the hormonal changes brought on by pregnancy, many women will experience more oil on the face. This truly annoying situation means skin can get clogged very easily with the products you used before you got pregnant. A great and inexpensive way to deal with this situation using things from your kitchen or medicine cabinet is by making a do-it-yourself mango mask.

Here we go: Mash one fresh mango into a soft pulp. Apply onto your face, leave for a few minutes, then rinse off.

Black Book Extra: If you want to spend a few extra dollars, use what many A-list stars reportedly use to keep their glamorous beauty routines all-natural from head to toe: organic and all-natural Jurlique. It's especially important for pregnant woman with fair skin and hair and sensitive skin to stay away from oil-based products.

A NEW VIEW

Our friend Elisabeth Hasselbeck on *The View* recently gave birth to baby number two but says it wasn't easy to get back into her skinny jeans two seconds after getting out of the hospital. "I couldn't believe it, but a press person asked: 'So, Elisabeth, what size were your jeans before the baby and what size are your jeans now?' I was like, 'Interview over!'" she jokes.

Elisabeth says, "It's a little annoying to push a person out and then all of a sudden you're required to be back to your perfect size in two weeks." She says it's all about accepting your new and changing body. "Everything is in a different geographical location now," she muses. A quick fashion tip: "Now I'm wearing the jeans that hurt me until through pure gravity they must stretch out and not hurt anymore."

Black Book Extra: We also got some advice from her *View* costar Sherri Shepherd, who jokes, "Just yesterday I said that I lost my baby weight. And my baby is two years old!" she quips.

ENVIRONMENTAL MAMA

You want to spread the word about living green to your unborn baby, but how when many of those stretchy pregnancy tops are made with such horrid, uncomfortable, and never biodegradable fabrics? We found a way that you can be stylish and organic at the same time. It's called MollyAnna maternity wear, and they have a great line of popular T-shirts in environmentally sustainable organic cotton. Stars such as Britney Spears, Jennifer Garner, Gwyneth Paltrow, Rachel Weisz, Angie Harmon, Michelle Williams, Molly Shannon, Michelle Branch, Tina Fey, and Brooke Shields are big fans because the duds promise it all. They're for those who are "bold, sassy, and preggo!" Trista Sutter of *The Bachelor* fame insists that she practically lived in MollyAnna "Body By Baby" and "I Can Grow People" T-shirts when she was pregnant with her little boy. It figures that stars love the soft, lightweight material. "They allowed people to know in a humorous way that I wasn't just fat. I wish they were appropriate to wear even when I wasn't pregnant," Trista says. We love the new organic line with all the hip and funny slogans such as "Birth control is for sissies" and "Coming soon to a hospital near you." There's even a new Daddy line with one shirt proclaiming: "It's all about DADitude. The shirts range from $36 to $38. Check out the line at mollyanna.com.

MAMA MILLA

Milla Jovovich, the gorgeous supermodel turned actress, is nine months pregnant when she talks to Black Book. Hide the peanut butter! "I'm happy to tell all the pregnant ladies out there that I've gone from 130 pounds to 193 pounds. It's a lot of weight to put on quickly, and I only have myself to blame," says Milla.

"I could eat peanut butter sandwiches and bagels all day. I see no problem with it," she laughs. "Of course, my doctor does see a problem with it. So I've gone cold turkey on the bread. I'm doing chicken and veggies and trying to be the healthiest mother.

"But if I could continue with the peanut butter, I'd be the happiest mom in the world!" she says with a laugh.

BB: How are you feeling today?

MJ: Honey, my bones seem soft now and my feet are killing me. All the physical training I've had to be a model and to do action films like *Resident Evil* really helps. So I strongly encourage women who are even thinking about getting pregnant to hit the gym before trying to conceive. It will still hurt to walk. No one tells you that part! But I can tell you that prior to conceiving, get in your optimum shape. You will be glad.

BB: How does a former model deal with the weight gain?

MJ: I don't mind, but my mom keeps bragging, "I didn't gain this much weight with YOU! I was skin and bones and just had a little bump." Yeah, thanks Mom! How helpful! I'm trying to deal with that and how gorgeous she was and how . . . get this . . . she even wore heels when she was pregnant with me. Now, my feet have grown three sizes. They don't tell you that part either. I can barely wear flip-flops.

BB: Are there any great beauty products that have gotten you through your pregnancy or just gave you a little pick-me-up?

MJ: I was shocked at how many friends sent me little beauty products. It's a wonderful thing that all women should do for their pregnant girlfriends because it's such a pick-me-up. Just buy them some creams or oils. What a great, inexpensive surprise that's so useful. I love anything from the company Mama Mio. They have wonderful stretch mark creams and amazing oils that smell so good. They also feel great, which is the most important thing.

BB: Do you have a favorite comfy outfit?

MJ: I haven't been able to get out of my stretchy empire-cut T-shirt dresses. Even with the weight gain those dresses drape perfectly and I feel good about myself. You don't want to wear anything tight.

BB: What are you looking forward to as your pregnancy comes to an end?

MJ: I can't wait to see my precious baby. And I'm going to have a whole appreciation of my old body! No more peanut butter!

Update: Milla gave birth to a precious baby girl she named Ever Gabo Anderson.

BEWARE OF YOUR FABRICS

When expecting, it's so easy to feel like a whale. The idea is that you want to do everything in your power not to look like . . . we won't say it again. We checked with costume designers at a few of the studios to see what tricks they use to hide or camouflage an expanding belly.

The experts agreed that you should always stay away from shiny fabrics no matter what Anna Wintour at *Vogue* says in the pages of the latest issue. Metallic may be trendy, but silks, satins, and sequins that show every lump and bulge and reflect light will draw attention to your increasing bulk, which is exactly what you don't want.

PREGNANCY SKIN CARE TIPS

When you're expecting you can also expect to slightly alter your skin care routine. Consider these tips:

- Start with a gentle cleanser. Use a nonresidue or glycerin-based facial cleanser. If your skin is ultra-dry, then try a soapless rinse-off cleanser that's mild and moisturizing. Wash your face no more than twice a day to prevent over-drying.

- Remember to moisturize with at least SPF 15 and with broad-spectrum protection (that works against both UVA and UVB rays).

- By the way, elevated hormone levels trigger the multiplication of pigment cells, which can cause facial blotchiness, or "the mask of pregnancy." Using sunscreen daily—even if it's thunderstorming outside—is the best way to avoid this nasty condition.

- If your skin is oily or you're breaking out in zits (usually worst during the first trimester of pregnancy), then ask your doc if you can use a product containing glycolic acid, alpha hydroxy acid, topical erythromycin (prescription only), or witch hazel.

- But stay way from topical retinoids (such as Retin-A or Differin) or salicylic acid. It's helpful to go into your cosmetics and check product labels for ingredients—it's best to use caution with these products and not use them when you're expecting.

- When you're putting on makeup during pregnancy, use a little less. It's not only a great way to shorten your morning routine when you're tired, but you don't need all those products clogging your new pregnancy oily skin.

- A foundation stick that doubles as concealer is great for covering under-eye circles and blemishes and for evening out skin tone. Chubby pencils are fabulous for smudging on eyes, lips, and cheeks, and they won't take up much room in your bag. If you're the kind of person who won't leave the house without lipstick, make sure it's moisturizing and contains sun protection. Finish up with a coat of washable, waterproof mascara and you're ready for the day.

SHOWER THE PEOPLE YOU LOVE

We're calling for showers in the 90210 zip code, and this is not a weather report. Baby showers are serious big business, and the deal is you have to top all the other expecting A-list mamas in town. To wit: Nicole Richie had a *Wizard of Oz*–themed shower at the Beverly Hills Hotel complete with a lot of Totos (the stuffed variety) and ruby red slippers as centerpieces. And yes, there was a yellow brick road with candy around it. Another one of our favorites had live butterflies released outdoors during her shower.

Beyoncé's little sis, Solange, had a baby shower with three hundred of her closest friends. Even the invites are swanky and hand delivered these days—with their pop-up designs, ribbons, and crystals, the invites go for up to $50 each.

We also love celebrity party planner Mindy Weiss's idea of taking four-ounce baby bottles and filling them with pink and blue jellybeans as table ornaments. Simply tie a pretty ribbon around the neck of each bottle and your guests will have a fun take-home gift. By the way, if you want to surprise everyone by announcing the sex of your baby, you can go all pink or all blue.

Make sure to bring a great gift to your important showers at the Four Seasons or Bev Wilshire. Jennifer Lopez's pre-baby wish list included a $3,495 Silver Cross Balmoral stroller, a $289 suede playmat, and a $349 cashmere outfit. Jessica Alba, Isla Fisher, Christina Aguilera, and Naomi Watts all had their wish list at the super chi-chi Bel Bambini in West Hollywood. They have a great $249 Svan high chair.

Kim Porter—mother of her and P. Diddy's twins—reportedly requested an $88,000 R-Class Mercedes-Benz for her registry back in 2006. No word if she got one.

MASSAGE MADNESS

Pregnant women often have aches and pains, and massage offers soothing relief—even if only temporarily. But what danger does massage hold for an expectant mother? According to Tony Deckard, a licensed massage and bodywork therapist from Asheville, North Carolina, the benefits of a massage during pregnancy far outweigh the risks.

"There is a theory that there are pressure points in the webbing of the hands and feet that can stimulate labor, especially during the later months," says Deckard. "Although this theory has not been concretely proven, it is best that these points be avoided. The abdomen is avoided simply for the mother's comfort, as the little ones usually don't like the massage and begin kicking, making Mom uncomfortable and unable to enjoy the massage. Otherwise, the only other contraindication of massage during pregnancy would be a complication in the pregnancy itself. But when done properly, a massage can be just what a pregnant woman needs to recharge and relax her overstressed body."

Perhaps it is the massage "tools of the trade" that pose the risk. Many massage therapists use oils and lotions during a session, but are they safe? "Massage oils used differ widely, but mainly those used are natural or herbal oils," says Deckard. "The only complication that I have encountered is when the smell of the oil, such as lavender, makes a pregnant woman ill. If this occurs, the oil should then be substituted with virgin, unscented oil. But the oils themselves pose no harm to either Mom or baby."

MANIC MANICURES

Many pregnant women find that their nails tend to grow more quickly, resulting in a need to groom them more often. What once was a biweekly visit becomes a weekly one. Visit any manicurist and you will see the finest collection of chemicals, from nail polish and removers to oils, paints, and skin treatments, all believed to be safe. But according to a recent report from the Food and Drug Administration, research indicates that chemicals in nail polish, nail polish removers, and the like, namely methyl methacrylate and acetonitrile (a chemical that breaks down into cyanide when swallowed), are in fact dangerous and can cause numerous health problems, including skin irritation, contact dermatitis, rashes, poisoning, and even death. These facts alone cause a concern.

But according to manicurist Heather Jacobson, it all depends upon the chemicals used—and who uses them. "Not all manicurists use the same products or use them in the same way," says Jacobson. "For example, I use mostly natural or biodegradable products, and the nail polish I use on my customers is 'edible.' It's not that you could eat it right from the bottle, but if you do ingest it—as most women do from time to time from biting their nails, licking their fingers, and so on—it won't harm you, as it has only natural ingredients. But others may still use products that contain chemicals that are not safe during pregnancy or otherwise. It's best to ask your manicurist or request that she use natural products. And if you're not sure, simply skip the nail polish and have your nails buffed for a natural shine."

ZITS THE PITS

There are some quick tips for reducing acne during pregnancy while protecting the health of your baby:

- Clean your skin to keep it oil-free during pregnancy.

- Use an oil absorbent microfiber cloth while washing your face to absorb the oil while gently cleaning.

- Keep your hands away from acne and rub gently while washing to avoid spreading bacteria to other parts of your body.

- Engage in daily exercise to increase blood circulation and flow, thus helping the skin to tone and stay healthy.

- Use lots of water while cleaning to control acne during pregnancy—this does away with icky leftover soap, which can result in collecting bacteria or irritating the skin.

- Take extra care not to rub near your outbreak, as it will smear the bacteria and you will get more zits.

- Wash fruits and vegetables before eating to remove herbicides, pesticides, and other chemicals that affect the growing baby and the health of your skin.

- Keep your skin dry and use an oil-free moisturizer five minutes after drying your skin.

Acne Treatment During Pregnancy: Our A-list skin care experts gave us a few tips to deal with acne during pregnancy:

- Use an astringent that is nonmedicated.

- Accutane, which is taken in the form of pills or tablets, is considered to be the best medication to treat acne. It is also known as Isotretinoin. You must ask your doc first.

- Tetracycline, which is an antibiotic, can be taken orally to treat respiratory infections and acne. Again, check in with your doc first.

- Apply an oil-free moisturizer.

BB EXPERT: BONNIE BELKNAP

From Kym: I met Bonnie Belknap when she was gathering all the products I needed to do segments with Ellen from our books *The Black Book of Hollywood Beauty Secrets* and *The Black Book of Hollywood Diet Secrets* on our favorite show, *The Ellen DeGeneres Show*.

For more than twenty-five years Bonnie Belknap has been one of the top food stylists/caterers in Hollywood. Her company, Gourmet Proppers, specializes in preparing on-camera prop food for film and TV as well as private catering for the stars. Bonnie has worked with and cooked for celebrities such as uberfather Brad Pitt, Harrison Ford, Madonna, Ellen DeGeneres, the cast of *Sex and the City*, Ben Stiller, Bruce Willis, the cast of *Friends*, Kate Hudson, John Travolta, Al Pacino, Will Smith, and Jada Pinkett-Smith, and new mom Jennifer Lopez.

She is a genius at accommodating the dietary restrictions of all these actors, so imagine what advice she can give us!

Contact Bonnie at gourmetproppers.com.

> **BB:** Bonnie, we know that you're supposed to eat healthy and cut the fats during pregnancy. Have you ever helped a client who had a fat-food craving do a favorite food in a better way?
>
> **Bonnie:** I do remember a client who loved fried chicken—the southern kind. She was preggers and had gained quite a bit of weight. Her doctor wanted her to cut back on the fat. I helped her marinate chicken in lowfat buttermilk and hot sauce. Then we tossed it in a bag filled with whole-wheat bread crumbs, a little whole-wheat flour, salt, pepper, and garlic powder. You shake off the excess crumbs and transfer to

a baking sheet that has been lightly sprayed with vegetable oil, then bake for one hour, turning to brown evenly. It's really easy to make, and no messy oils. My client loved it. In fact, her husband also loved it and it helped him get rid of the weight he was gaining during her pregnancy.

BB: Is there an alternative to the greasy pizza that many women crave during pregnancy?

Bonnie: I came up with this one on a movie I was working on. One of the lead actresses was pregnant and everyone was eating pizza in this scene. To cut the fat, I took long, thin Italian breadsticks and wrapped them with either thinly sliced ham or turkey, then dipped them in marinara sauce. It's quick, easy to eat, and a much healthier snack than pizza.

BB: What is your favorite healthy snack for pregnant woman?

Bonnie: My favorite anytime snack for pregnant women is what I call nature's fruit pops. They're great to suck on when nauseated: Skewer two or three fresh grapes on a wooden skewer, which is about four to five inches in length. Freeze them and then serve them plain or dip into nonfat yogurt.

AND NOW A FEW WORDS FROM BOBBI BROWN

Even when you run a multimillion dollar cosmetics business like Bobbi Brown Cosmetics (a 50 million dollar business), it's still about the kids. Bobbi Brown, forty-one, is wife to Steven

Plofker, a lawyer and real estate developer, and mom to sons Dylan, eight, and Dakota, five.

What are her best makeup tips for pregnant women? "I like to recommend that pregnant women keep their beauty routine simple and easy," says Brown. Her list of essentials includes a concealer for blotchy or uneven areas and dark under-eye circles, yellow-toned foundation (which Brown swears is best for all skin types), a pink blush, and your favorite lip color. For best results, Brown recommends first putting on concealer (one shade lighter than your foundation) just where it seems necessary, because that may be all you need. Then apply foundation, but only on the areas without concealer. Doubling up just cancels out the effect of the concealer, she says.

What about the days when you have two seconds to get ready? "Blush is the best way to give yourself a boost," says Brown. Her signature technique is to apply a bronzer or skin tone blush across the whole cheek as a base and then a splash of pink right on the "apple" for a natural, I-just-finished-exercising look. Pregnant women can also give themselves a beauty and mood boost by spritzing on a clean, fresh scent. Choose something light and pretty, says Brown, since your sense of smell is heightened during pregnancy.

THE CELEBRITY NEW MOMS' TIME-SAVING BEAUTY SECRET

Many of the celebrities we've interviewed here at Black Book HQ tell us that this is their best-kept beauty secret: laser permanent hair removal. It's why they say they feel free to take their kids to a last-minute pool party or jump into the Olympic-sized drink at Angie and Brad's French abode with the kids during baby swim lessons or head to the beach in Malibu to hang with Courteney and David with a moment's notice. Laser permanent means no stopping to shave, wax, or feel self-conscious or uncomfortable about ingrown hairs in the bikini area. Amen to that, everyone. It also means that harried moms don't have to figure out how to keep the little guys and gals quiet at the chi-chi salon while they go in for their monthly wax and rip, which is always so pleasant. (Hi, I'm Tonya, your waxer. You: Hey, Tonya, nice weather we're having . . . owww-wwwww. Toyna: Did that hurt? You [thinking]: "No, ripping hair out of my privates is the most fun I've had since giving birth.")

The BB spoke with Ronda Hawara-Nofal, owner and founder of Blue Medi Spa in Sherman Oaks, California. Nofal says permanent laser hair removal is the long-awaited answer for expecting or new mothers with ingrown hairs (goes so well with water retention) and women who are tired of shaving because of the time-consuming aspect of it and the burden of staying on every little hair. It's also very popular for celeb women, who get the laser as soon as they find out they're pregnant because they don't want to have to deal with the pain and inconvenience of waxing or shaving. This also ensures that on delivery day they will be groomed, hair free, and ready for the big arrival in more ways than one.

What about the pain and the price? The bikini and underarms—the most popular procedure among the expecting stars—are about as painful as waxing according to actress and *Dancing with the Stars'* Shannon Elizabeth, who is a big fan, says Nofal. In fact, she has had her bikini, underarms, and legs done, and loves it. The prices include a package of three sessions for $400 and afterward at a cost of $100 a session. For underarms it's even more affordable, for a package of three sessions for $300 and after that $75 per session. You will need three to six treatments, depending on the color and texture of your hair, and the sessions should be scheduled six to eight weeks apart.

Nofal reports that women actually come back to her spa after the laser hair removal crying, telling her thank you and that it changed their life. Once you have a newborn, literally every second counts, so laser gives you more time with your new bundle of joy. Blue Skin Medi Spa is at 14622 Ventura Boulevard, Sherman Oaks, California, 91403, 818-783-3600, bluespa .com. You can check out comparable laser hair removal spas in your area.

SPECIAL DELIVERY GOWNS

Celebrities don't like to do anything in the normal way and must upgrade when it comes to what they wear while giving birth. No, Chanel and Gucci aren't allowed even at Cedar-Sinai. But you can do something about those horrible hospital gowns even if you don't live in the 90210 area code. A company called dearjohnnies has solved the problem. Celebrities such as Marcia Cross, Jenny Garth, Brooke Shields, Tori Spelling, Mariska Hargitay, and Samantha Harris all wore their own personalized, monogrammed dearjohnnies custom-made hospital gowns for delivering their own special deliveries. They even have snap-downs for breast-feeding and snap flaps for special medical attention. They also snap down the back and are super-duper soft while keeping mom's famous behind covered up. Hospital staff appreciate that the new moms are wearing a regulation hospital gown. It's a way to be glam and comfortable during labor and in the days that follow. The moms love the super-soft fabric and loose-fitting designs. These gowns are made of 100 percent cotton and are trimmed in gorgeous ribbons to make the new mom feel better about herself after popping out their little costar. Check it out at dearjohn nies.com.

ONE HOT MAMA

In Hollywood having children is "IN." Looking like you've had children is "OUT." That's why Verabella in Beverly Hills offers a high-priced skin-care treatment called the Hot Mama Facial ($155). With chilies and herbs, be warned it is NOT for mothers to be but for after you have the baby. The name actually comes from one of the ingredients . . . ready? It's from human placenta from Russia, which is harvested, sterilized, and freeze dried (excuse us, we have morning sickness and we're not even pregnant) and then put into a fleece mask. The fleece is then activated by water, and when placed on the face makes the new mother's tried, stretched, and drained skin firm and supple. By the way, firm and supple are always "IN."

MIRA, MIRA, ON THE WALL . . .

Academy Award–winning actress Mira Sorvino has starred in *Mighty Aphrodite*, *Beautiful Girls*, and *Romy and Michele's High School Reunion*. The New Jersey native is the daughter of actor Paul Sorvino and Mom to Mattea, three, and Johnny, one, with actor hubby Christopher Backus.

BB: You've had two children in the past three years. Tell us about that.

MS: I was pregnant for eighteen months over three years and have given birth twice in two years. You could say I'm a little bit tired!

BB: Eighteen months is a long time. What little things did you do during this time to make yourself feel prettier?

MS: It gets hard the bigger you get. There are days when you think nothing will make you feel better today! What helped me the most was getting cute clothing. The maternity clothing made me feel so depressed. I kept thinking, "How can I possibly be attractive to my husband in a tent!"

BB: Did you figure out any secrets?

MS: Yes, and this was crucial. I would go into the large-size women's stores and get clothing in 14s or even 16s. Women can get 1X and 2X if they need. It's so fantastic because you can find beautiful clothes and you feel feminine. These clothes are made out of great material and they look sexy. There is even some feminine frilliness to some of them, and that made me feel so great.

BB: So you felt sexier?

MS: I just wanted to feel like a girl and not a house! I swear, during this time I started to think I should start an attractive clothing line for pregnant women—design it with custom fabric, and make sure it breathes. I don't understand why some of the standard maternity wear is made out of this scratchy fabric that never breathes. Why not just use cotton! I'd also love to see some vintage clothing in pregnancy wear. That would be so pretty!

BB: How did you lose the weight after your kids were born?

MS: It took me a long time to lose the weight after my second child was born. I did a lot of running in Central Park with my double baby jogger. It's the best workout, hands down. You run with this double stroller with two kids in it. That's about seventy pounds of kids and stroller to push while you run. I also tried to run at the same pace as the other runners. This was just the best calorie burner, and the weight fell off.

My mother was the most beautiful woman I ever saw. All I am I owe to my mother. I attribute all my success in life to the moral, intellectual, and physical education I received from her.   —George Washington

YOU AIN'T HEAVY, YOU'RE GIVING SHILOH A BROTHER

When you're pregnant, it's a great equalizer because no matter if you're Angelina Jolie or Queen Latifah, Soleil Moon Frye or Nicole Kidman, it's hard to look good when you are quickly adding upward of twenty, thirty, or forty pounds onto your frame. Here are a few top celebrity stylist tricks culled by Black Book for looking your best when you are at your heaviest.

- Oversized bags subtract inches from the hips: Did you realize that even though you don't have a diaper bag yet, you can start camouflaging your growing belly with a large handbag? According to stylist Julie Weiss, a gigantic purse slims any figure—when hugged against the torso it can make the body appear more lithe and delicate in contrast. By the same token, you'll want to remember that a small bag can make a woman appear larger.

- Tunics camouflage belly bulge: It doesn't matter if it's Tory Burch, Talbots, or Target, just invest in long tops— they are one of today's fashion staples. According to Weiss, there is a key to finding the most flattering tunic. Make sure it's loose enough to hide the expanding hips and belly but not so long or thick that it adds bulk to the hips and thighs. The ideal length: The hem should hit your wrists when your hands are at your sides.

Hoops distract from flaws: We always wondered why girls like Kim Kardashian can be caught without makeup but never without their big hoop earrings on. Well, now we know: Weiss says that oversized hoop and chandelier earrings aren't just stylish, but they're also a smart way to appear leaner. Big earrings bring emphasis to the face and away from your growing figure. Talk about hoop dreams.

Our favorite pregnancy T-shirt quote: "Spare Me Your Birth Story"

SLEEP LIKE A BABY, YOU BABE

You're pregnant, you're XL, you're uncomfortable, and now it's hard to get any sleep, so you're one grumpy mama-to-be. The answer can be as easy as five minutes and the cost is low: Run to your local flower shop and pick up a bunch of inexpensive Gerber daisies. In a study from Queens Medical Center in England, higher levels of atmospheric oxygen were found to stabilize breathing and increase the duration of sleep by 10 percent. While most plants absorb carbon dioxide and give off oxygen during the day, the Gerber daisy does the process at night, ensuring that you will—pardon the pun—sleep like a baby!

BB EXPERT: LORI ANN ROBINSON

Lori Ann Robinson is a Hollywood image and fashion consultant as well as a four-time Emmy-nominated costume designer, author, and professional speaker. She has worked with Hollywood's most beautiful moms-to-be as well as up-and-coming and established professionals for more than twenty years. Lori has designed for many celebrity moms-to-be, including Tracey Bregman, Katherine Kelly Lang, Hunter Tylo, and Genie Francis on TV shows including *The Bold and the Beautiful* and *General Hospital*.

Lori is truly an expert in maternity dressing, having worked with four pregnant actresses at one time—on one show! She is also the spokesperson for TC Fine Shapewear, a division of Cupid Intimates. Visit Lori at larconsultants.com or e-mail her at lori@larconsultants.com. We dished with her an all matters baby.

What are the biggest beauty secrets women can use during their pregnancy?

The biggest beauty secret is finding clothes that keep you looking and feeling your very best. I have worked with many pregnant actresses. At one time while I was designing *The Bold and the Beautiful*, there were three pregnancies, and none of the actresses was actually supposed to be pregnant on the show. Lots of smoke and mirrors to camouflage. One of things that I really tried to do was keep the actress feeling beautiful in her clothes. There are so many regular-size fashions out there that are conducive to maternity wear. Very often regular-size clothes can be bought, just a couple of sizes up. Women often wait until the last few months to wear traditional maternity clothes.

How do you look like you lost the weight after giving birth and going back to work when you haven't lost the weight?

The best way to camouflage post-pregnancy is with fabulous shapewear. Shapewear can reduce lumps and bumps after the baby. Not only will it smooth you out and mold your shape, but it is terrifically supportive for your midsection and back. Shapewear has come a long way, baby—it's not your grandma's girdles anymore. I love the brand TC Fine Shapewear. The fabric is so light and comfortable . . . and it breathes! It never rolls down or rides up. It is an actress's post-pregnancy biggest secret.

What is the best piece of advice you received about pregnancy and looking good and professional and put together when you aren't feeling that way?

You can have a few key neutral pieces and to add that "punch." Keep colorful jewelry and scarves up around your face. The eye is drawn to bright and light colors. Change out your accessories, which will always fit and will enable you to get more mileage out of repeat dressing. Build a small-capsule wardrobe where all pieces will mix and match with each other.

At the Black Book, we want to tell moms how to do a Five-Minute Mom Makeover. In five to ten minutes what can a harried mom do to look good?

My tips: No one wants to see those maternity clothes ever again after the baby. Plan a post-pregnancy wardrobe before the birth. You do not need to live in unshapely sweats. You want to look your best even when exhausted. There are many items of clothing on the market with stretch that are comfortable and washable. Mix and match pieces that you can wear before you return to your normal size.

LOW PRICE, HIGH-END MATERNITY FASHIONS

We got this insider fashion trick from baseball great Steve Garvey's wife, Candace. Years ago when Kym was pregnant with her son, Hunter, she was doing a show called *Home & Family* with Christina Ferrare and Chuck Woolery. "I was getting bigger by the moment and found myself with numerous invites to lots of black tie, red carpet events with my husband for the Daytime Emmys, Soap Opera Digest Awards, and so on. With my growing belly, I couldn't afford to purchase the high-priced designer gowns that I would wear once and never wear again," Kym says.

"Candace pulled me aside and told me to do what all the celebrity wives, socialites, and stars do when they are with child. They head incognito to the designer resale shops!" According to insiders, the Hollywood ladies go there to purchase Dior, Chanel, and Bottega at rock-bottom prices and in double-digit sizes that they will never see again after the baby is born.

So that is how they look so great in such gorgeous dresses without breaking the bank.

UNDERCOVER AGENTS, WE ARE

When you're expecting a baby, you can also expect your entire body to be hot and sweaty. (How Gwen copes with this in front of Gavin, the world will never know.) Well, we have a tip for the luscious one: There is a special underwear that absorbs sweat but is water resistant and great for those hot days when private places need to be dry and cool. T. Santiago makes underwear from a unique absorbent cotton exclusively from South America. This fiber makes the items not only water resistant but also sweat absorbent. The sexy underwear dries almost instantly and shapes to the body perfectly while wet.

Find them at tsantiago.com.

BODY BY BABY (AND SAMMY)

When you're having a baby, it's hard to think you could have a body, too! Sammy's is one of the best workout wear stores in Beverly Hills, a staple for fitness buffs and Hollywood stars alike. Owner Sammy Shakerchi says in Hollywood when you're having a baby it doesn't mean you can stop taking care of your body. According to Sammy, one of the most popular clothing pieces among pregnant customers is the One Step Ahead workout pant, at $44. It's not just the feel, comfort, and durability of this pant; it's the drawstring. According to Sammy, who can't keep them in the store, it's the most comfortable and nonbinding workout gear for mothers to be, and it's safe for the baby she is carrying because there is no tightness, tugging, or pressure on the belly. Women buy them fourteen at a time and we can see why—they stretch so beautifully, fit everybody perfectly, and last forever so before, during, and after baby you will always have the perfect workout pant.

Available at Sammy's, 453 Beverly Drive, Beverly Hills, California, 90210, 310-246-0376.

BB EXPERT: ROXANNE BECKFORD HOGE

Roxanne Beckford Hoge is the creator of the onehotmama .com Web site, one of the most popular places celebrities go to find out all things cool, hip, and informational in the mothering arena. She's also an actress, sure, but in Los Angeles, that's hardly unusual. (Her husband, Robert Hoge, is also an actor.)

Roxanne has four children and has found parenting to be challenging, annoying, life-changing, exasperating, and wonderful, and probably a whole lot of other adjectives, too.

Roxanne got her B.A. in psychology from Davidson College in North Carolina, and then promptly threw herself into the world of corporate public relations for Citibank and the Rouse Company. An early midlife crisis precipitated a move to Los Angeles and the never-forgotten world of acting. She's been a working actress since the early 1990s, doing television, film, voice-over, and commercial work, in addition to enjoying several years onstage with an improvisational comedy troupe. Since starting her adventures in motherhood, Roxanne has written for Salon.com as well as for her Web site and breast feeding.com, and is currently working on adding film clips to her site with lots of tips for moms on the run.

What makes her worth listening to? She's had children, both with and without drugs. She's had twins. She had trouble nursing and tried to go back to work within hours of delivery. She stayed home. She's done it all, and unlike most "experts," she has a real laboratory with four live children.

BB: Please tell us about your tricks and secret wardrobe tips to not show when you're showing if you're an actress or a working woman who doesn't want to reveal her pregnancy just yet.

RBH: Ah, yes, the hiding of pregnancy. I've done it so many times I do feel like a specialist. Please, if you are a pregnant teen reading this, give it up. Run, don't walk, to your mom and spill the beans. Okay, for all you women in jobs or situations where you just don't feel it's anyone's business that you're pregnant, take it from me: It can be done. When I was pregnant with the twins, I had been scheduled to work on the movie *Bewitched*. I could not find a way to tell Nora Ephron that I would be growing on a daily basis, and my part was being filmed over the course of five weeks. That's a lifetime in a twin pregnancy. The Lord intervened and the schedule somehow shifted to just three weeks. This made my wearing Spanx, control-top panty hose, AND a girdle a little bit more bearable. That's a little extreme, but just so you know, it did not damage the babies. My wardrobe was the tiniest, tightest (thankfully stretch) skirt and sweater and sky-high Marc Jacobs heels. I suggest the following instead: Don't wear anything clingy. Keep all your clothes that have structure in rotation—tailored jackets you can wear open, for example. Play up your neckline with a deep V collar (with lapel). You'll find that those dress shirts start to strain, first across the bust and then across the belly, so find some one size up with draping or wrapping. Keep your old suit pants on as long as possible by looping a rubber band around the button, through the buttonhole, and back again. Black (and other dark color) velvet absorbs the light, so use that as a shirt/belly material whenever possible. T&L. Tits and legs—show these and most men will skip right over the burgeoning belly. (This tip also works postpartum to great effect!)

BB: What was your biggest feel-good secret during your pregnancy?

RBH: Gosh, I'd have to say, after three pregnancies that went a total of 116 weeks, the number-one trick is to pull a Fernando (remember him from *Saturday Night Live*? "To look good is to feel good and I feel marvelous!!"). Now, I'm not an exceptionally vain woman. I generally go from shower to car (without kids) in thirty minutes. But I really believe that if you slouch and keep your PJs on all day, you'll end up feeling like you look, which will be crap. So, during a SIX-WEEK, doctor-mandated, hospital-monitored bed rest for my first baby (and this is before the days of wireless Internet connection, mind you), I got up every day and used my allotted ten vertical minutes to get dressed into something cute. That first pregnancy was RIGHT on the cusp of the introduction of body-conscious clothes. I had gotten hand-me-down stuff from a fashionable friend with gobs of money, and they were HORRID. Tons of overall-type blousy things. I found stretchy tops and slim-cut long skirts and lived in those—and I remember my shrink (my shrink!) asking if perhaps I was ambivalent about being pregnant because I wasn't wearing regular maternity clothes (i.e., tents). The other biggest feel-good secret is getting in shape. Now, here's the scoop. I'm not now and never have been a regular workout person. It's sporadic, if at all. But I made time for regular prenatal Kundalini yoga during all three pregnancies and swam every single day with the twins. (And I hate water—frizzy, naturally curly hair doesn't do well in the YMCA pool room.)

BB: What was your biggest beauty secret during your pregnancy?

RBH: Looking and feeling good go a long way to helping you on off days. I will never get the "I'm wearing my husband's sweat clothes" or "Just buy bigger sizes" school of dressing pregnant—both just make you look fat! And say what you will about how great it is for people to come in all sizes and shapes, when you look fatter than you ARE, it'll make you feel awful. I also learned from dear Vicki Iovine *(The Girlfriends' Guide to Pregnancy)* to NOT lop off all my hair, and trust me, I wanted to—I have had two children in the dead of Los Angeles summers. But you need to think proportions—your belly is HUGE, so even it out with as much hair as you can (sans spray) and well-cut bottoms that have a little presence. And I felt that I (and other preggo chicks) was glowing—so play it up. I swear, I got hit on so much when I was fully pregnant. Enjoy your new shape and the life within and your fabulous skin (after the first-trimester zits leave). It's so sexy.

I also got massages and chiropractic adjustments—I'm not a large person, and the weight was pretty darned hard on my hips and back.

BB: What couldn't you live without during your pregnancy?

RBH: I went through buckets of Mamatoto cocoa oil sticks with the first two kids, and then the Body Shop discontinued them. Drat! But I did lube up my considerable girth every single night during all three pregnancies, and I have no stretch marks on my belly, even though I have them other places from puberty weight gain. Fun tip for second-time moms—my son and daughter used to oil my belly for me as their nighttime job.

I lived in the Perfect Pant by Dress (onehotmama .com carries it) and wore them so much that I got another pair just the other day, with no future pregnancies in sight. They are just awesome—a fleecy microfiber that can be casual or dressy, no waistband so your belly is always the perfect size for them, and a slightly wide leg to even out whatever's going on . . . on top.

During my pregnancies the Spaghetti Tank from Belly Basics was the only tank with a built-in bra, but now everyone makes them. We have a great inexpensive one that I'd use now as my uniform layering piece to still get wear out of my regular clothes and to help tuck in that outtie belly button you get at the end (by the way, I used scotch tape or Band-Aids to avoid having that protruding out of all my fab cotton/lycra outfits near the end).

Also, I could not handle my regular underwire bras—not only because they didn't fit, but also because you start the day one size and end up way bigger in the rib cage! What's that about? So, although they're a little pedestrian looking, I ended up reaching for my Bravado nursing bra a lot—they have an extra-wide elastic rib band instead of underwire. This expanding rib cage is another reason to live in Spaghetti Tanks.

My maternity swimsuits were fabulous—I had three or four the last go-around because the best thing in a multiple pregnancy is to swim as much as you can. But this is the one item of clothing you cannot fudge. You might feel like your regular nonmaternity suit fits "fine," but the crotch is pulling up and making your choice of wax clear to everyone else around the pool. Trust me.

What I would have ten of if I got pregnant again is Bella Bands—they're basically stretchy tubes of fabric that you can use in the beginning to hold up your old pants (back in the day, I used the loop-a-rubber-band-through-the-button-hole trick), in the middle to cover your belly when you're wearing nonmaternity tops, and after the baby to cover your mummy tummy while you're nursing.

Mama Spanx—no need to explain—but if you think your undies crawl up your crack now, just wait till you're seven months along.

The last item is nonspecific but truly necessary—a collection (large or small) of clothes that fit, that make you feel pretty, and that look as good as they feel. Think of pregnancy like a round-the-world cruise—you want to pack your favorite things.

BB: What were your pregnancy cravings?

RBH: Gosh, for some reason I ate a lot of lamb with the first two babies. The twins were a whole different kettle of fish. Early weight gain (unlike in a singleton pregnancy) is correlated with fuller-term, higher-birth-weight babies, which I really wanted. The goal is more or less twenty pounds by twenty weeks. Eating becomes a real job, a chore almost, because you have to eat when you're NOT hungry. And anything I felt like eating filled me up after two bites, thanks to the double tushies resting on my stomach, so I lost my usual love of food with them. I ended up craving physical movement and release—like swimming and yoga—because I was so heavy and unwieldy.

BB: How did you lose the weight after giving birth?

RBH: Nurse. Nurse early and often. Nurse on cue and eat well, which I do anyway, and the weight will do what it wants to do. I have to say, I have had four children and gotten to know a zillion hot mamas thanks to schools and our Web site, and it is very rare that people don't end up getting back, pretty much, to the way they looked before. Women who were round before are round after, and people who were athletically built before are athletically built after, and so on. It's just that not everything is necessarily in the same place. Even if you have a C-section, surprise! No one will have told your pelvis, which dutifully used the hormone relaxin to expand and widen during the end of your pregnancy. It ain't snapping back overnight! More important than actually losing the weight (which you will—everyone will—the moment you give birth. Just baby and placenta ought to be good for ten pounds or so, so step on a scale and rejoice in your superior metabolism) is to (see above) look like you have. In other words, if you get back into your husband's sweats or the fat clothes that passed for maternity clothes, what will be your motivation to move your butt? Nothing. But even if you're wearing nicely cut maternity jeans five months postpartum (like I have—I LOVED those jeans!), you will not forget they are maternity jeans. And you will look good, and people will tell you that you look good, and then you'll feel rewarded and keep on that path. I never dieted because I nursed so much, and you need lots of calories to make milk! But I've always eaten good food, and I do have the added benefit of being allergic to wheat. So if I want a pie, I've gotta make the crust from scratch—can't do the McDonald's apple pie. So that forces me to eat homemade and to get my burgers protein style (wrapped in lettuce instead of a bun) and never to have pizza. I also almost never used a stroller for anything but stuff (until I had twins), so I carried my babies in a sling wherever I went. That's aerobic exercise PLUS weight-bearing from doing the grocery shopping.

BB: As a mom who certainly is busy, how do you take care of yourself? Any quick tips for beauty, diet, or exercise as a mom? Any stress relievers?

RBH: Taking care of yourself can sometimes feel like something you have to add to your already overloaded list of things to multitask, but if you live as mindfully as you can, making dinner for your family can feel like a vacation (not on the nights when everyone is screaming and there's nothing in the larder/pantry, but on a regular day). Here are my wishes for every new mother (and even the old ones)—do not waste a moment of time whining about how you used to get to do this or that or what you'd be doing if someone wasn't hanging off your breasts at this very moment. I wasted a lot of beautiful time doing just that with my first baby (it is, after all, the biggest adjustment), and it took three more babies to get really good at it. The first thing is, enjoy your babymoon. Not the trendy new term for a prebaby vacation (although that's certainly fun), but declare to everyone that you will be nuzzling someone's little neck for the first three months after birth (six for my twins) and they are to leave you alone. The irony is that I "accomplished" more with this attitude than with the back-to-auditioning with my THREE-WEEK-OLD first baby. What a nut! When you are comfortable in your job as mum, that's when you can move mountains. That said, as you get closer to delivery, have a pedicure and one last bikini wax if you're allowed. The sight of me pregnant with twins getting up on that table will be talked about by the Russian waxers at Raya Taver for years to come. Get a hairdo that will last— with Cameron (bed-rest baby) I used the time to try out cornrows/extensions—where else was I going? And with the last three I tried to time blow-outs for every few days so that I'd be ready for the photo fest that comes with having newborns.

If you can get to a postnatal exercise class that includes baby, do it. You'll make friends who actually have babies and remember what it's like (trust me, even for a semi-pro like me, the fog of war creeps in and you might even wax rhapsodic about middle-of-the-night feeding when you just want sympathy about them) and your instructor/guru will understand if you stop to nurse during class. My yoga teacher noticed, however, that I was always nudging baby awake during ab work, and finally banned me from waking up the baby the moment she started a leg-and-arm-lift series. Once they're toddling around and it's too hard to get out, I am a big believer in TiVo, DIRECTTV, and, for the old-fashioned, tapes and DVDs. Don't have to leave the house. Half an hour and it's over, and if you can do it most days, you're on the right path. Hey, do you see celebs appearing at LA Fitness postpartum? No. A private trainer is what they use. If you can do that, great, but Denise Austin is free and on TV every morning at 7 a.m.

My biggest beauty tip is to buy a beauty magazine without any babies in it. Do this after your babymoon and *at least three times a year* thereafter. Why? Because fashion and beauty are not static, and time will have passed you by. These magazines will help you to realize that most of the things in your under-the-bed storage box (where you put your unpregnant clothes) are now woefully out of style. Toss those things (to Goodwill, of course). How to survive the sartorial challenges of the first six months? Well, remember what I told you about how to dress on the way up to your due date? Reverse it. Of course, you'll want some new clothes—nursing clothes have come a LONG way from the schmattes I encountered over ten years ago, but even a great nursing shirt needs to be paired with pants or a skirt. What to buy? Nothing expensive. Even if you have gobs of money, get your postpartum pants and skirts at Forever 21 or other knockoff discounters. They won't last forever, thus saving you the temptation to stay that new (bigger) size for*ever*. (Got that tip from my first-ever babysitter.)

My favorite part of being an actress is hair and makeup. Okay, truth be told, it's craft services, but after that it's the time with the artists in the makeup trailer. Here is the number-one reason why celebrity moms don't look so, well, mom-ish. Someone tries the new makeup and hair looks on them periodically. Seriously, that's the big one (the other big reason is lack of invisibility, but more on that later). If you had a baby in the late 1990s, like I did, and you were a trendy, well put-together young (or not so young) thing, you used Mac or Laura Mercier and you had the neutral/natural look down with a side of dark brown lipliner and nude lipstick. Fast-forward ten years. That look is OVER, and if you haven't had the good fortune to be on a movie set, you will be frozen in time (my friend Anita calls it the wedding day/prom night face). After the third and fourth babies, when I'd taken a hiatus from on-camera work for a bit, I realized things needed updating and booked a lesson with a makeup artist. You can also get tips in department stores for free. I can't say enough about this. Look like you belong in this decade.

So here's my last point about this, and then I'll get off my soapbox. The other big reason that celeb moms look so great is because they avoid the one thing that happens to every new mother that is so dangerous to her self-esteem and, thus, her look: With a new baby and a slightly poochy tummy and all the gear you're now slogging around, you are invisible. You walk through the mall to get a break from all the crying, and everywhere around you are pretty young things without any drool on their shirts and the stores are full of things you can't wear. It becomes easier to shop for baby because you know his size will fit him and you not only don't have time to get into a fitting room, you don't want to see your soft, flabby tummy and your budget may be a little tight and who are you without your job/career/high heels and silk dress anyway? You're still you. And you still deserve to look like you. Our point over at OneHotMama is that if you nurse for a year you're saving your family almost TWO GRAND!! Spend a little on yourself, honey. That'll relieve some stress. That, and sex with your husband, but ONLY if you've sorted out birth control, because the fear of another pregnancy after you've had a taste of reality is very unsexy.

I have so much more to say (as you can imagine), but I need to move on because I MUST get to bed before someone wakes up!

BB: What was the one item, food, clothing, or ritual that helped you get through your pregnancy the most?

RBH: Pregnancies one and two, I'd have to say my swimsuits because the babies were born in July and August in LA. Although I also swam every day with my twins. So maybe movement is the one thing.

BB: What is the best piece of advice you received about pregnancy and mothering?

RBH: It's actually something I picked up at a La Leche League meeting, where I went when I was desperate for help and companionship. It was "This, too, will pass." And it does. All the bad stuff eventually changes, but so does the good stuff, so hold on when you can. My babies have now all lost their baby smells.

BB: What is the best piece of advice you can give about pregnancy and mothering?

RBH: Be aware. Of how you feel, how you look, how your baby feels inside you and out. How what you say and do matters—deeply—to another human being. So feel and notice everything you can.

BB: What was the absolute biggest, fattest lie about pregnancy or motherhood that is perpetuated and should be exposed?

RBH: Gosh—it's a bit harder to lie about stuff because there's so much info out there. I guess for me it was really a lie about womanhood. That lie was that we are just like men. And then that fantasy collided with the reality that *I* was pregnant, *I* gave birth, and *I* was producing milk from my body. It was an ugly adjustment. We get to experience the most amazing miracles—of birth and caretaking—and we shouldn't ignore that or think less of it because it's women doing it. It's what feminists fought for—the realization that this is valuable work. And work it is—no violins and dreamy soft focus here. There are a LOT of bodily fluids involved.

BB: How do you feel about the pressure new moms seem to have nowadays—to look perfect, lose the baby weight, and get back to work five minutes after having a child?

RBH: Oh, that was so me with my first and second babies. I wanted to get BACK. But you need to go forward. It's going to be a brave new trip, and you'll cobble together the way you make it work the best you can, and it'll look different for every woman. But get off your own back. We are our own harshest critics.

Want to look perfect, lose the weight, and get back to work in five minutes? Have lipstick in your hospital bag, wear a fabulous colored top, and say hello to your new boss—the baby!

BB: What is the BEST part about being pregnant and being a mother?

RBH: For me, for about one glorious year, it's that I get to control another human being (evil laugh). Then they begin to roll over, and it's never the same again. The very best part is seeing that you are capable of heights you never imagined, and that these little creatures are entrusted to us almost wholly formed. Really, we can screw them up, but as I have four, I've gotten to see four very different, very unique souls from day one. What a privilege that has been.

Overheard in a Beverly Hills Delivery Room: One starlet was so afraid of those cheeky paparazzi that she insisted her gardener drive her to the delivery room. She hid out in the backseat of his old Ford truck with an old blanket over her head just to avoid the shutterbugs getting any snaps of her when her water broke. Yes, she walked into Cedars with leaves and grass clipping falling from her hair and shirt, but she didn't care. Talk about going green.

CHAPTER 3

Mommy Needs an Eyelash Curler

Post-Preggers Body, Face, Hair, and All That Good Stuff

I gained sixty pounds and I'm proud of it. Why do I need to watch my weight when I am pregnant?

—**Our hero and mentor, Kate Hudson**

Hi Nursing Moms,

We love you and appreciate how tough it is now to look at all those girls in strappy little tank tops and no bras. Under normal circumstances we give those girls little headshakes, and not because we hate them. Okay, we're jealous. But the point here is if you're nursing, please, pretty pretty please, check with your doctor or nursing specialist before trying any of the foods or shakes or tricks or tips in this chapter. We don't have medical degrees, and what works for one star might end up to be D-list for your efforts and for your new bundle of joy. By the way, we can safely say that you should make your husband get up in the middle of the night to do a few feedings. We can't think of any doc in the world who would be against that one. And meanwhile, you can get some much-needed rest and dream of George Clooney. Oh, sorry. You're a new mother now and you should be dreaming of things like bottles, diapers, and Brad Pitt in a bathing suit on a beach somewhere in the South Seas.

XOXO,

Kym and Cindy

Did you know . . . the average amount of weight women gain during pregnancy is thirty pounds: one or two pounds in your breasts, six to eight pounds with the baby, one to two pounds with the placenta, and two to three pounds of fluids. The rest of the weight is in increased blood and a calorie bank that your body maintains for the baby.

YOU CAN GLOAT: NO BLOAT

Bloating and water retention are two of the biggest battles women fight while pregnant, so we found that celebrities were drinking large amounts of a new type of tea post-birth that's hitting Hollywood in a big way and may be a great way to help with the water and bloating. Tulsi Tea (Holy Basil Tea) is known as the queen of herbs in Ayurvedic medicine according to Hollywood A-list skin-care expert Tracie Martyn, who handles the faces of Madonna, Renée Zellweger, and Kate Winslet. Sip this tea whenever you have the time to relax. Tulsi Tea is said to reduce inflammation, and who needs to be more inflamed when she is pregnant? It costs only $4.99 at Whole Foods.

A-LIST MOM: TORI TORI TORI

Oh, Donna!

Ask the down-to-earth, lovely Tori Spelling for a little motherhood advice and the former Donna Martin from *Beverly*

Hills, 90210 just giggles and pats her nine-month-pregnant belly. "Oh my God! Other mothers probably have better advice that they could give me than I have for them!" she says.

"I can tell you that my son is so heavy he's an arm weight," she jokes.

Tori has done a fine job with adorable toddler Liam and recently gave birth to a darling baby daughter named Stella. "How do I handle it all?" she says. "I'll tell you my secrets. You need to have a hands-on dad who has a great connection with the mother. Then you're really a team and it's not just one of you but both of you who are doing the parenting." In addition to late-night feedings and the terrible twos, Spelling also has her hit reality series with her actor husband, Dean McDermott, and several bestselling books.

BB: Tell us more about how Dean is so hands-on with the kids. We hear from a lot of moms who complain that they really have to beg their husbands—again and again and again—to help.

TS: Dean is more than hands-on. He is so unbelievable with Liam, and that really helped when I was pregnant with our daughter. At the end it was so hard to do anything simple like carry Liam. I didn't have to ask Dean. He just carried the baby. It's so great when you don't have to ask. We're also very lucky. One of the best things is that we work together on our reality series. We get to take our babies to work every day, which is really amazing because we get to be with our children every single day. It's a unique situation and we're very fortunate.

BB: Congratulations on being pregnant for the second time. Do you have any tips for pregnant women? Any cravings?

Dean: Sorry to butt in. She did send me out for Rocky Road ice cream a few times.

TS: The only craving I've had has been Rocky Road ice cream, but that tapered off. The first pregnancy my one and only craving was for a root beer float. I don't get really bad cravings. You hear about these crazy cravings that pregnant women get, but I never had that. Like I never wanted to eat dirt or anything.

BB: Do you have a nanny?

TS: We're doing it without our nanny, Patsy, these days, which means we're doing it alone. Patsy wasn't actually a nanny. She was a baby nurse who came on our show and into our lives. She was supposed to be with us for two weeks but stayed a lot longer. She stayed nine months because we all just fell in love with each other. She became family more than anything else and we loved having her with us. But it was time for her to move on and do other jobs as a baby nurse. Liam was already a toddler by then and it was just the three of us. Soon it would just be the four of us.

BB: How did you prepare Liam for baby number two?

TS: Well, he was a little too young to be able to understand that there was another baby coming. But I kept showing him my belly and I kept saying "baby." At one point when I would just point to my belly, he would say "baby." I'm still not sure he understood what it all meant.

BB: You did a great job losing the weight after Liam. Any advice?

TS: I was on NutriSystem and it was definitely a challenge at first. I didn't think I'd have a problem dropping weight. I've never had any weight issues. But honestly it was difficult, and I found myself having to go on a diet program and really stick with it after I had Liam. By the way, it worked great and then as soon as the weight came off I got pregnant again.

EAT TO LIVE, EAT TO LOSE

To lose the baby weight, it's all about calories in and calories out. If you're not breast-feeding, top LA docs tell us women who want to shed the pounds should stick to about 2,000 calories a day, but every bite must count. A good way to get in those calories while staying healthy and getting max energy for taking those 2 a.m. feedings on with gusto:

- Breakfast: Cereal, milk, fruit, and orange juice
- Lunch: Grilled chicken or tuna on salad or mixed greens
- Dinner: Pasta, a protein, and mixed veggies
- Snacks: Yogurt, fruit, milk

Again, the point is every bite should make you stop and say, "Is this nutritious? Am I feeding myself in order to take care of myself?" If you find yourself eating a candy bar, the answer must be no.

(Although an occasional cheat along the way can maintain your mental health.) Docs tell us that you do need to add extra calories if you're breast-feeding (and please check with your medical professional or breast-feeding counselor). As for exercise, with your doc's approval, walking is a great mild way to get back into the action.

BB EXPERT: LISA CHASE, FOUNDER OF CELEBRITYEVERYTHING.COM

"It's all about affordable luxuries for moms and dads," says the fabulous Lisa Chase, a radio star in her own right and founder of the ultra-hip Web site CelebrityEverything.com. Lisa, who is a contributing writer for the *New York Daily News* and *Hampton Sheet*, debuted the site in 2007. Lisa has also been writing about and interviewing celebrities at *Star*, *Celebrity Living*, and *Life & Style* magazines since 2004. CelebrityEverything .com is the ultimate one-stop resource for catching up on the daily scoops and trends, as well as all the beauty items, fashions/accessories, spas, and mom products that celebrities love!

We picked Lisa's brain for the best products for new moms (and even a few new dads).

BB: Do you feel for the celebrity moms who are hounded to lose the weight in record time?

LC: It's so hard for the new moms because there is a tremendous amount of pressure in Hollywood to bounce back from having a baby in just weeks. Yes, these women can hire trainers and get the delivery meals. That helps. But it's also hard when the paparazzi are just waiting to snap one little patch of cellulite. And if you're the average mom out there, you don't need this to trickle down and have the whole world think, "Why can't I bounce back like Halle Berry?"

BB: You sell products on your Web site that celebs use. What is a favorite for both new moms and dads?

LC: I love a product called EShave Cream. Courteney Cox uses it for her legs and her husband, David Arquette, uses it on his face. Your face and legs feel like a baby's butt. Courteney loves the citrus kind. Men like the cucumber cream, which is crafted for sensitive skin. Courteney shows a lot of leg on *Dirt*, so it must be working! I even told my doorman in New York City about this product and he told the other doorman. The first feature of a doorman clients see is his face.

BB: Any tips for a harried, young new mother that a famous harried young mother is using these days?

LC: Nicole Richie says that she loves to put on false eyelashes. They cost nothing, and it makes her feel more alive and awake. It's a great tip because false eyelashes are simple, you can buy them anywhere, and it's just a little bit of glamour to make a new mom feel special.

BB: That's a great tip. Can you give us a few others?

LC: Stars who are new moms also like Couvrance, a corrective makeup. It's a little green stick that takes care of any redness. It's awesome because it can really even out your skin after giving birth.

BB: Are there any great gift tips for new moms that you've heard from Hollywood?

LC: The trend now is moms sharing beauty products with their babies. Moms use certain products on their babies and it smells so good that they think, "I gotta have that because I want to use it myself." One of the most coveted products is Noodle and Boo French-Milled Baby Soap. It's one of the best baby soaps ever. I had Noodle and Boo send me some, and my husband had no idea that suddenly he was using baby soap. When it was all done I was like, "Honey, do you like it?" He said, "Yes, what kind of soap is it?" I said, "It's called Noodle and Boo." My husband said,

"Well, it's French milled." Katie Holmes and Britney Spears use it. The shampoo is also fantastic.

BB: We hear you have some Sarah Jessica Parker scoop?

LC: An interesting scoop is that I heard Sarah brought an Alora Ambiance Reed Diffuser into the delivery room to defuse and disinfect the air. There is one that has a duck on the front of it and it's just so cute. The latest obsession is what do I pack in my bag to go to the delivery room. This is a great idea.

BB: Now there is nothing that makes any woman—recently pregnant, currently pregnant, or just someone who had too many carbs that day—feel better about life than a great spa treatment. What are the mom stars into these days?

LC: There are so many fabulous spas out there. I know Liv Tyler does facials and manicures at Bliss Spa in New York City. But here's something else all new moms love: their hot milk and almond pedicure. After those all-nighters with the baby this can really make you feel better. It's also a great idea for pregnant women . . . when you get to the point where you can't see your toes, it helps to have someone pamper your toes. You should treat yourself and feel better. Mariska Hargitay also goes there. Kate Hudson gets deep tissue massages at Bliss. These keep a mommy's stress down. Angela Bassett goes to the Mamie Skin Care Center in New York City for facials. It was her husband, Courtney Vance, who got her into facials. He was taking care of his skin there. I always give props to the men who get treatments and realize that the women in their lives need one, too. Angela also travels a lot. As a mom on the go, she knows a tub of shea butter works so well when you're traveling. It's so good on dry skin. Your skin just drinks it right up.

BB: Do you have a model mom tip?

LC: Kate Moss walked into a photo shoot and a fashion editor screamed at her, "Whatever she has on her face I must have it." It was BioElements, and models love this brand because they're moisturizing nuts. It's the best, and Demi Moore is apparently a fan as well. These women do have phenomenal skin.

BB: Do you have a few good stretch pointers?

LC: Samantha Harris of *Dancing with the Stars* used cocoa butter all over her tummy to get rid of stretch marks.

Black Book Extra: We also love the entire BellaMama line for stretch marks.

BB: Having a great diaper bag is all the rage in Hollywood. What are the best ones out there right now?

LC: My big tip to moms who want to look cool is to get a fabulous diaper bag. Heidi Klum has a rockin' leather motorcycle bag with black leather and metal studs. It's so hot, and it's by a company called Nest. Jennifer Lopez has a metallic diaper bag from Kale. The point is all of these moms have something special. They don't carry these big dowdy diaper bags from years ago. They don't carry bags your husband wouldn't touch with a ten-foot pole. I love the Web site poshtots.com. It's filled with high-end products including all sorts of celebrity stuff and daddy diaper bags. Jack Black has one that looks like a really cool daddy backpack. It's manly and it doesn't look like a purse.

And it's good for Dad to have his own bag. Dad needs his own bag and a different bottle. This way Dad's bag for baby can stay packed so he can go off with the baby and you can go to the spa for a treatment. There is no excuse that he isn't prepared to take the baby for a few hours.

Black Book Extra: We also love the Nest Whipstitch Leather Diaper Bag in Platinum, which is also a favorite among the stars. You will be the envy of all the really cool mommies at the sandbox.

BB: What is the best post-preggers workout tip you've heard from a new mom?

LC: We heard that to lose the baby weight Jennifer Garner did a program with interval training. She would run for a minute, rest a minute, run for two minutes, rest for two minutes. You just keep it going and kick it up or down depending on how you feel. It's a cool way to jolt your body and rev your metabolism.

BB: Do you have a favorite celeb post-baby weight-loss story?

LC: I loved that Elizabeth Hurley admitted she holed herself up at Elton John's mansion after giving birth to her son. She said that all she ate was fish, veggies, and rice. I love that Liz didn't say, "Look, I magically lost this weight." She said, "This is hard and I'm doing it the old-fashioned way with protein and veggies." I also like that Catherine Zeta-Jones admitted she did a low-carbs post-baby diet.

Hollywood Speak: Hub-Manservant—This is a husband who doesn't really work or have anything to do but just trails after the famed wife and the kiddies. Example: "She

never has to worry about hiring a new nanny because she
has that fab hub-manservant on the home front."

POST-BABY DIET TIPS AND RUMORS FROM MOMS WE LOVE

- To get in shape before the Spice Girls world tour, Victoria Beckham was reported to drink two pints of seaweed shakes a day! High in fiber and low in fat, Posh found the shakes were a great way to fill her up.

- Becoming a mum can do strange things to people. Many A-list actresses control calorie intake by eating jars of baby food after giving birth.

- Flowers at your table will make you eat more, even though the smell may clash with the smell of your meal. We love all those friends who sent flowers, but keep them in your bedroom and not your kitchen!

HAIR APPARENT TO DEMI AND GWYNETH

One of the main things pregnant women complain to us about is the damage having a child does to your once luscious locks. When you're pregnant most likely you will not have a lot of extra time to be running to the hair salon for follicle masks and intensive conditioning treatments to get your hair back to its original shine before you became a mommy-to-be. If you yearn for Demi's shiny hair or Gwyneth's long strong locks, then why not try this tip to help repair and add shine to your locks while you're at home feeling ready to pop or getting ready to nap with the baby.

Shine-Boosting Hair Care
for New Moms

1 egg yolk
2 tablespoons mayonnaise
2 tablespoons olive oil
1 avocado

Combine all the ingredients in a bowl. Apply the mixture to dry hair, cover with a shower cap or plastic, and let sit for fifteen minutes. Rinse, and your hair will be as luscious as when you were a bambino.

BABY BUTT FACE

If you're having a baby, you might as well ask the doctor to save you a little of the placenta (afterbirth) while she is down you know where because human placenta has become the high-priced-must-have-anti-aging-face-lift-without-the-knife-wonder-cream-of-Hollywood. Even one of those Desperate Housewives says she uses it and loves it.

The makers of EMK Placental skin care products in Beverly Hills tell us the results are in indisputable, that it firms, lifts, and hydrates the skin better than anything else around.

Black Book Extra: If you are a real hard-core beauty aficionado, then this may be the trick for you. There have been rumors around Hollywood for years that aging starlets have resorted to flying to Switzerland and Germany to go to expensive spa and anti-aging clinics to have injections filled with alleged sheep placenta, all in the quest for everlasting youth and beauty. Well, Hollywood took heed, and we hear that placenta creams are flying off the shelves as the newest way to fight wrinkles and preserve the face. By the way . . . the unique biological compounds in placenta ensure that the fetus is supplied with the necessary nutrients and oxygen needed for successful growth. Placenta purifies the mother's blood of hazardous toxins before it enters the embryo and provides the embryo with all the nourishment it needs for existence, growth, and defense from external risk factors.

On your skin, it's being called a face-lift without surgery.

Overheard in a Beverly Hills Delivery Room: One supermodel had an ultra-swanky baby shower on the roof of a major LA hotel. The only problem was it was 100-plus degrees up there on a hot summer afternoon and the other models—who of course were only nibbling on air as a food group—began to pass out in droves from the heat. The preggers one just popped a few tarts and told the other gasping models that she didn't care because the minute the baby was born she was going back to total starvation.

CHAPTER 4

Stars Losing It (We Mean the Weight)

I love being pregnant, which is why I've done it four times. I love feeling the baby kick. Then you give birth and there is so much pressure. —**Tracey Gold**

I felt like my body wasn't mine. I didn't put any judgment on myself. It was a beautiful time. —**Elizabeth Hurley**

Instead of hitting up the Governor's Ball or any other party, we opted for sweats and In-N-Out Burgers. Being preggers kind of takes the fun out of partying until the wee hours. Sleep always sounded better to me. —**Jessica Alba**

BE A PUSHER

Sometimes it's good to push—good for your waistline. The American Council on Exercise just completed a study of how many calories moms burn when they push a stroller! To find out how many calories you burn, exercise scientists at the

University of Wisconsin La Cross had women push baby strollers that were thirty-five pounds in total weight. Basically, that's a one-year child plus the diaper bag. The moms walked three miles per hour and burned 6.2 calories each minute. That means if you push the baby for an hour, you will burn 372 calories! That's actually more calories burned than riding an exercise bike at the gym for ten miles an hour for your standard twenty to thirty minutes or for even doing that boring twenty-minute slow jog on your treadmill. In fact, an hour outside with your baby moving around burns a small meal. Just remember to thank junior one day for helping you get into your skinny jeans.

Hollywood Speak: Carb Resting—It's a far nicer way of saying that post-birth you're giving up the bagels and biscuits. Instead of telling the world that you're on a boring low-carb diet, it sounds much more chic to say, "No, I didn't delve into the bread basket at the Ivy. I'm carb resting."

BB EXPERT: CYNTHIA PASQUELLA

Cynthia Pasquella is one of Hollywood's favorite nutritionists. She is a respected certified clinical nutritionist, wellness coach, fitness expert, detox specialist, and media personality. She is also a certified aerobics instructor and personal trainer.

Cynthia's clientele includes professionals, celebrity actors, models, athletes, and soccer moms! As a former model, actress, and fitness competitor, Cynthia saw firsthand the lengths that people will go to in order to lose weight. Rather than succumb to the pressures of starving and crash dieting, she looked for a healthy way to stay slim and tone while still being healthy. She found it in a program of balanced nutrition and mind and body detoxification.

Cynthia practices an all-natural mind-body approach to weight loss that gives you the results you want without the stress, inconvenience, and harsh side effects of most diet programs.

Cynthia is currently working with a world-renowned herbal supplement company to create a line of all-natural, organic bath and beauty products. She continues her hosting career in television and is a guest favorite of many radio shows. She also counsels Elisha Cuthbert, Robert Downey Jr., Shannon Elizabeth, Kate Beckinsale, and Brooke Burke.

BB: Tell us a little bit about your philosophy when it comes to new moms, babies, and eating routines.

CP: Hold on to your ovaries, ladies, because you won't believe some of the things I have to share with you!

Now more than ever it's crucial for you to start your children's life with healthy foods. It's not just for your children, but this goes for you, too! It's more than just eating healthy; it's truly about creating a healthy lifestyle for your family. I know you've heard this a million times before, but let me share some things with you that I bet you haven't heard to better put things into perspective. Take a simple head of lettuce today. You go to the grocery store, pick it up, take it home, and eat it thinking you've made a healthy choice. Well, you made a better choice, but did you know that it would take fifty of those heads of lettuce that you just bought to equal the nutrient levels found in just one head of lettuce fifty years ago? That's a pretty big difference, isn't it? You can thank herbicides, pesticides, and chemically laced fertilizers for that. By their nature these chemicals are meant to kill, and they do . . . they also kill the nutrients that crops receive from the soil.

Make it a point to purchase organic fruits, vegetables, and meats. For those of you who may not know, "organically grown" means grown without the use of any harmful chemicals such as pesticides. Many fruits and vegetables actually absorb those chemicals into their skins, which you then ingest. If you haven't tasted organic fruits and veggies, then you need to go to the store right now! They're full of rich, vibrant flavors and smells. You can just taste the nutrients and health they're bringing into your body!

But it's not just the food we put in our bodies that we have to watch out for these days. Have you ever been stressed out to the point of saying "I might need to see somebody about this"? Are you thinking of getting a prescription that can help destress you? Don't waste your time or money. Just stop drinking your tap water. Recent studies indicate that many prescription medications, including antibiotics, anticonvulsants, mood stabilizers, and sex hormones, are in your drinking water. These medications are synthetic compounds that spread throughout your body, and their residue can lodge itself in your tissues and stay there for years. Water-processing plants hurl all sorts of chemicals at this to "clean" the water, but because of the potency of these compounds, they can end right back in your glass. Some experts believe that these prescription drugs can cause significant changes in the human body, including hormonal imbalances. If you're reading this book, then chances are you know a little something about hormones being out of whack! It's not a good thing!

The solution is to filter your water, but there are so many water filtration systems on the market. It can be something as simple as running out to Target and buying a Brita pitcher. Don't waste your time and money on bottled water because the majority of the bottled waters out there use plain old tap water anyway, and most bottled water is packaged in plastics that have been shown to leak a chemical called BPA, or Bisphenol A. BPA is an endocrine disruptor that particularly affects developing cells. So fetuses and children, whose organs, brains, and reproductive systems are still growing and changing, may be most at risk. In adults even small doses of this chemical can cause enlarged prostate, altered mammary glands, genetic damage to eggs, changes to reproductive organs, accelerated puberty, reduced fertility, and altered brain development. Many manufacturers of plastic baby bottles, such as BornFree and Green to Grow, have now created bottles without this harmful chemical to help protect your little one. By the way, Nicole Richie received the Green to Grow bottles at her baby shower and just fell in love with them.

Not quite convinced that healthy foods grown without chemicals and filtered drinking water are necessary? Well, maybe this will help you change your mind. In 2003, the Environmental Protection Agency (EPA) released a study that examined the umbilical cords of randomly selected babies from varying backgrounds. The results were astounding and quite scary. The study found a whopping 287 toxins in the newborn's umbilical cord blood. Of these, 180 cause cancer in humans or animals, 217 are toxic to the brain or nervous system, and 208 cause birth defects or abnormal development in animals. Scientists refer to the presence of such toxins as "body burden."

Even though some of these chemicals may not show harmful effects immediately, subtle changes in development can show up later in childhood as learning or behavior problems or in adulthood as cancer or neuro-degenerative disease. According to the EPA, many diseases have been on the increase over the last thirty years: asthma (100 percent increase from 1982 to 1993), childhood brain cancer (40 percent increase from 1973 to 1994), acute lymphocytic leukemia (62 percent increase from 1973 to 1999), and autism (1,000 percent increase from the early 1980s to 1996). Early life exposure to environmental toxins is one of the main suspects of this increase.

Pretty scary, huh? I know that's probably enough to convince you to take steps toward leading a healthier lifestyle, but just in case, here are a few more reasons. If you're wondering what other harmful toxins are floating around out there under your nose, just take a look at your bath, body, and personal care products. Seriously, I mean it. Due to gaping loopholes in federal law, companies can put virtually any ingredient into personal care products. Even worse, the government does not require premarket safety tests for any of them. If you see ingredients such as thimerosal (a big word for mercury), lead acetate, petrolatum, mineral oil, paraffin, hydroquinone, sodium laurel sulfate, 1,4-Dioxane, polyethylene, polyethylene glycol (PEG), polyoxyethylene, "-eth" ingredients (such as sodium laureth sulfate), methylparaben, propylparaben, ethylparaben, and butylparaben, then don't use it. These chemicals are have been linked to numerous diseases and conditions, including breast and other cancers and birth defects.

As a mother or mother-to-be, a chemical group you want to be especially cautious of is phthalates (pronounced THA-lates). These are plasticizing chemicals that are probable human reproductive or developmental toxins and endocrine disruptors. They cause reproductive birth defects in laboratory animals, particularly males. Two phthalates often used in cosmetics (dibutyl phthalate and diethylhexyl phthalate) have been banned in the European Union. Unfortunately, phthalates are still found in some nail polishes and hair sprays and are commonly hidden on ingredient labels under the term "fragrance." *Yes, fragrance.* I highly recommend that you steer clear of products with fragrance, and this warning is especially for pregnant women, babies, and pubescent young adults.

So, what's a mom to do when she needs beauty products without sacrificing her health? Go to your neighborhood health food store, a Whole Foods, or even Target (they've recently started carrying natural and organic product lines) for your beauty and personal care purchases. But be careful because again the labeling on bath and body products is loosely—and I mean loosely—controlled. Make sure you read all the ingredients on the label to look out for synthetic chemicals that have been added. A wonderful company out there called Dr. Bronners recently tested some so-called natural and organic products, only to find these products in fact contained a number of synthetic harmful chemicals! See why I tell you to read the label carefully? SoCal Cleanse (socal cleanse.com/shop) has an excellent line of organic soaps and bath and personal care products that are completely safe for both you and your little one. Their activated charcoal soaps are not only made with certified organic ingredients, but the charcoal works to help pull harmful toxins from your largest organ—your skin. Considering your skin can absorb up to 60 percent of your daily toxin intake, it's truly one of the best products out there.

For more information or to test your own beauty products for dangerous toxins, check out Skin Deep at cosmetics database.com. This is a huge database sponsored by a nonprofit group that lists the ingredients in more than 25,000 popular products and whether they're safe for you.

BB: Is that really so important? And is it costly?

CP: People always tend to ask this question because it does seem like it's so much more expensive to eat organic and purchase organic products. In reality, it isn't at all. Many more grocery stores stock organic foods now, making the price much more affordable and very close to their non-organic counterparts. In addition, there are so many farmers' markets that offer delicious organic foods and products that are grown and made locally for very reasonable prices. On average, you can expect to pay approximately 15 percent more for organic foods. This is a small price to avoid fats, sugars, and chemicals that can lead to heart disease, cancer, diabetes, hormone disruption, and obesity. You also won't have to worry about paying for medications for these conditions later on. This applies not only to food but all organic products. For example, when I started using charcoal soap to cleanse my face and body, I stopped having to see my dermatologist and no longer had to purchase skin care medication for acne and other problems. That's well worth the $10 to $15 per bar! Plus, it lasts forever!

If you want to include some organic foods into your diet but don't want to pay the higher prices for all the fruits and veggies you buy, then there are a few smart buys. These are the foods to make sure you get organic: strawberries, bell peppers, spinach, cherries, peaches, cantaloupe, celery, apples, apricots, green beans, grapes, and cucumbers. These foods tend to be higher in pesticides than others, even after washing. To find organic food buying groups, co-ops, health food stores, local retail farms, and farmers markets' in your area, visit local harvest.org.

BB: Give us some of your suggestions and tips on what the celebs eat before, during, and after pregnancy.

CP: It's so important for you to be aware of the fact that just because you're pregnant, it doesn't mean that you can or should eat anything and everything in sight! Many people, celebrities included, do this very thing and then have a hard time getting the weight off later. Please keep in mind that the food you're putting into your body is meant to nourish the little one inside you, so you want to make sure you're making healthy choices. I recommend a diet of organic fruits and vegetables, whole grains, and lean proteins that are also rich in omega-3 and omega-6 fatty acids. A great way to sneak in your omega-3 and omega-6 fatty acids is by drinking hemp protein shakes or using hemp oil on foods such as salads. Hemp contains more EFAs than flax oil and provides the perfect three to one EFA balance. It is also free of potential toxic contaminants commonly found in fish oil supplements. I've also heard of several celebrities using hemp oil on their tummies to prevent stretch marks, and it works like a charm!

Nicole Richie was a fan of hemp protein shakes and also ate a ton of organic and vegetarian food while she was pregnant with Harlow. Gwen Stefani also loved to munch on organic veggies and would sip organic tea throughout the day during both of her pregnancies. Angelina Jolie insisted on eating nothing but organic foods during her pregnancy with Shiloh. And, of course, these diet choices seem to have paid off. All of these mothers had wonderful pregnancies and were back down to their prebaby weight in no time.

BB: What is your number-one tip for losing the baby weight?

CP: As a nutritionist, I see so many people who want the pregnancy pounds to drop off super-fast. Well, it took you nine months to put on the weight, so it might take you a little time and effort to get them back off again. Heidi Klum said it best: "I always think, 'Look at how people were before they were pregnant. If you were a toned, healthy, energetic person, most likely you will be like that again. You can't kid yourself.'" Don't you just love her?

The first thing that I recommend for all my clients looking to lose the baby weight, celebrity or not, is to start with a good detox program. It's wonderful for jump-starting a healthy nutrition and fitness lifestyle and can prepare your body for shedding the pounds fast by increasing your metabolism so you can burn fat more efficiently. Denise Richards detoxed using SoCal Cleanse—an all-natural product that contains wonderful organic herbs like ginger, cinnamon, dandelion, and green tea—after giving birth to her two girls, and she looks amazing! Gwyneth Paltrow is a fan of the peppermint and hibyscus SoCal Cleanse Organic Detox Teas.

I even recommend that every woman detox before getting pregnant because the toxins in your body can penetrate the placenta and enter through the bloodstreams of both you and your baby. As we've already seen from the study done by the Environmental Protection Agency, with an average of 287 toxins being found in the umbilical cord of newborns, it's imperative that you take the necessary steps to prevent this. If you plan to become pregnant, detox at least two months before you conceive.

One word of caution: You should not detox *while*

you're pregnant or breast-feeding. Doing so can pass the toxins you're excreting on to your baby through the umbilical cord or breast milk. Detox before you get pregnant, after you finish breast-feeding, or, better yet, both!

BB: We hear that you know a few insider tips about Angelina Jolie wanting to detox her system . . . to perhaps prep for baby? Tell us about that.

CP: Overall health is so important to Angelina, especially now that she has this growing, not to mention beautiful, family. She was a big fan of detoxing and did a full cleanse using SoCal Cleanse Detox Formula and Organic Detox Teas before she got pregnant with the twins. Obviously it was a good step because she's ready to give birth soon and is absolutely glowing! She's truly the picture of a healthy expectant mother!

Hollywood Speak: Sandbox Socialites—When you're the wife of a powerful mogul who shuns the nanny every once in a while to actually take your own child to the park. You sit with the other mothers whose names are often in bold face in the society pages and can be heard saying, "I have to go to the Butterfly Ball for World Peace later tonight and my dress is . . . wait . . . Allegra, please stop picking your nose on the teeter-totter. We'll never get you into a good preschool if you keep this booger action up."

BODY BY HALLE BERRY

Halle Berry is our hero for many reasons, including the fact that she's a talented artist, Oscar winner, and world-class beauty. We're also admiring how she got her body back in Berry-tastic shape after giving birth to baby Nahla Ariela

Aubry. Berry hired a celebrity trainer named Ramona Braganza, who has also put Jessica Alba and Anne Hathaway through the paces to fitness glory. Berry's secret to getting back in shape was a commitment to hitting the gym one hour a day, five days a week. Specifically, Berry split her workout between three cardio segments, including the elliptical, kickboxing, and stairs. She also climbed a few hills and added strength training with an emphasis on leg exercises and, of course, ab work. The results can be seen in every magazine around. As for her diet, Berry is diabetic, so she has always been careful about what passes those gorgeous lips. "I eat a lot of veggies, lean protein, and complex carbs," Berry says. "I'm also drinking water, and lots of it."

BODY BY ELISABETH

There was a lot less to view when Elisabeth Hasselbeck had her son and then seemed to morph back into prebaby shape. She says that after giving birth to son Taylor it wasn't easy to get back into top shape but she did it. Her secret? She focused on running and weight training after her doc gave her the okay, with ab work added to the mix twice a week. Even better is her mental outlook on weight because Elisabeth says that it's not just about being the hottest mama at the playground but about having a strong and positive attitude about her appearance, which will then set a great example for her daughter Grace. She says, "Body image has nothing to do with scale numbers, it's how you feel inside. This is the first time I've felt free from that, because I am working out in a way where I feel so strong that there's no room for those doubts."

BODY BY MADGE

After giving birth to Lourdes and Rocco, Madonna still defies gravity! Her trainer, Tracy Anderson, says that anyone can keep up with Madge (we wish) in the bod department if you just keep mixing up your workouts. The same routine, she insists, limits muscle building and toning.

Her workout includes: Run for one song, skip with another, and sprint (or go a little faster) with another on your treadmill for a total of thirty minutes. Do 10 reps (working up to 100) of each of the below:

- Arm Raises. Stand with your feet shoulder-width apart, and, holding three-pound weights, lift your arms together into a V above your head. Lower your arms and repeat. Keep your wrists and elbows a bit bent.

- Single Arm Pulses. Grab those three-pound weights, lift one arm holding the weight above your head, elbow bent, and then straighten out the arm. Repeat on the other side.

- Ballet Grand Pliés. Stand up straight, heels together, toes a bit apart. Bend at the knees and go as low as feels comfortable, and then return to standing position.

- Abdominal Crunches. While lying on your back, place your legs out in front of you and put your hands on your sides. Keeping your legs straight, lift up to do a crunch, and then release.

Anderson has a new DVD out called *Dance Aerobics*, which helps you burn the fat fast and tone muscles.

Black Book Extra: Anderson says that you should never use weights that are heavier than three pounds, and you should try to work out six days a week for thirty minutes.

Overheard in a Beverly Hills Delivery Room: What major movie star with the gorgeous blond locks was afraid of coloring her hair during her recent pregnancy? It wasn't that she was worried about the controversy over using hair dye chemicals but that the paparazzi would have spies at her salon who would report her for the color job. In order to get past this annoyance, she insisted that her colorist not only come to her home to do the dye job, but she also made her sign a confidentiality agreement!

A FEW MORE SLIM MAMA TIPS

1. Aloe vera juice can help you lose weight after having a baby, but we tried it, and if you can get it down, you are a better woman than we at BB Land.

2. Seaweed—you see it at the beach, and it's actually really good for you. It's not just because of Victoria Beckham. It is no accident that the longest living people on earth are the Japanese, and experts say that's because they make seaweed an important part of their diet. Studies show that it binds toxins in the body and flushes them through the system. Scientists even found that it helps prevent breast, endometrial, and ovarian cancers. So put a little seaweed in the blender and make a shake: At BB HQ we hear that all the skinny girls drink it in the morning. It helps curb their appetite and sweet cravings and it's very high in antioxidants.

3. If you're in a "why not, it might work and can't hurt" mood, then try blue-tinted sunglasses: Not only does your food look gross through blue-tinted glasses, but it actually raises the serotonin in your brain, which has been linked to blue light. Serotonin has been connected with various effects on mood, sleep, and appetite. MAO inhibitors, which reduce the breakdown of natural serotonin, are often used to treat depression. This trend started when handsome hunk Johnny Depp was spotted donning blue-tinted sunglasses all the time. A few paparazzi or TMZ decided to research it and to everyone's surprise found out that there are in fact studies that show that wearing blue-tinted sunglasses can help aid in weight loss. Hey, if you're buying a new pair of sunglasses for summer anyway, why not make them blue?

A QUICK POST-PREGGERS TIP

Did you know that popcorn plus oatmeal equals a flat tummy? Yes, it's true that whole grains help, but let's back up a bit. You've just had that gorgeous baby, and the area you're focused on is your not-yet-flat tummy. A great way to melt tummy fat is with whole grains. Researchers compared two groups of dieters—one that ate whole grain foods and another that avoided whole grains altogether. The dieters consumed the same number of calories, but the ones who ate the whole grains shed more fat from their midsection than those who didn't eat them.

A-LIST MOMMY: SALMA HAYEK

"It's the best time in my life to have a baby because I've done so much, and now I can really focus on motherhood," says Salma Hayek, mother of gorgeous infant Valentina.

"One doctor told me it was a boy. I really wanted a girl, and I knew it was a girl. Then when she was born I was so happy she was a girl," Salma says.

"A lot of people ask me where the name Valentina came

from. I wanted her name to have meaning. Valentina means courageous one," Hayek says. "One night I got very nervous about that name, though, and thought that she was going to be a revolutionary."

Is she spoiled? "She is so spoiled, and I will not apologize for it," says the actress.

As for getting back in shape, Salma says, "It was so hard because I gained a lot of weight and had gestational diabetes. The pregnancy was hard. As soon as the baby was out, like many other new moms, I thought 'I'll just lose the weight. I'll breast-feed and it will fall off.' Everybody tells you that if you breast-feed the weight will disappear.

"It's a lie! It's not true!" she cries. "The only reason people lose weight is if they're not eating and they're breast-feeding. And this is not good for the baby."

Hayek took a more sensible approach to getting rid of the weight. "They tell you it takes nine months to get it and nine months to lose it. I'm taking my time. I've lost most of the weight now. I lost slow and did that through working out. The rest will go when it's time to go."

DRINK TO SHRINK

We have found a great anti-bloat water to help flatten your tummy after you have the baby. Mix a little bit of ginger, cucumber, lemon, and spearmint leaves (to taste, you can experiment) in an 8-ounce glass of water. Stir and enjoy watching your stomach deflate.

SEAWEED FOR YOU, NOT TWO

Yvonne Bishop Weston is a nutritionist and founder of Foods for Life. When asked to comment on Victoria Beckham's new seaweed and algae diet that has helped her look so svelte after three babies, Weston explained that a diet with seaweed in it is not as crazy as it sounds.

"Algae and seaweed are superfoods with many of the vital nutrients your body needs. Seaweeds and algae such as chlorella aid detoxification, help reduce water retention, and break down fat deposits. In addition to being a useful weight management tool, seaweeds and algae can be an excellent skin treatment, even helping with problems such as acne," Yvonne told *Look* magazine.

Yvonne says she often uses seaweed and algae shakes for clients at her Harley Street nutrition clinic. "Particularly if people are aiming for weight loss but have a hectic lifestyle and are struggling to fit three nutritious meals and two healthy snacks into their day," Yvonne reveals. "Victoria is using algae and seaweed shakes as part of a personalized nutrition strategy."

For more information or to buy algae and seaweed shakes with chlorella algae and dulse seaweed, go to optimumnutritionists.com.

Black Book Extra: Superfoods such as chlorella algae, seaweed, and hemp protein are also turning out to be great weight-loss helpers, as are hemp oil and hemp seeds. But to get the best value out of your investment in these foods you should make at least one appointment with a qualified nutritionist to optimize your diet, check for existing deficiencies or digestive absorption problems, and determine a personalized strategy. This will save you money in the long run, and you will see how long-term stress can thwart your attempts at weight management even given these diet aids. Optimizing your digestive system is the key, and stress can be counterproductive.

CHAPTER 5

Your Little Costars and You

Being a parent is my first job. It's what is most important to me. —**Sarah Jessica Parker**

The moment a child is born, the mother is also born. She never existed before. The woman existed, but the mother, never. A mother is something absolutely new.

—**Rajneesh**

KATIE HOLMES DOES THE DEPOT

She's dressed in de la Renta, dripping with diamonds, and defined by the latest Suri hairstyle. But when you want to find the real Katie Holmes you have to go to one of her favorite stores. "I know how to push a cart at Home Depot," says Mrs. Tom Cruise. "I'm not a wimpy girl. I can push a super-heavy cart. I've been to the Depot many times with the other moms."

Naturally, there will be photo ops when Holmes checks out new crown molding. In her suite at the Casa Del Mar Hotel on

the beach in Santa Monica, California (a favorite major celeb
hideaway), the tall, slim Holmes just smiles without flinching.
She's dressed in black Oscar de la Renta creased pants and a
starched white blouse (also from Oscar). Her glossy brown hair
is in a short bob with fringed bangs and her eyes are wide but
determined. Mrs. C is one tough mama.

BB: Have you gone through the terrible twos with Suri yet?

KH: I've never met a two-year-old who is terrible. I have a lot of
       nieces and nephews and cousins who were babes. I'm from
       Ohio. We have a lot of kids. So I have yet to meet a terrible
       two. I'm so cool with every stage my daughter goes through.
       I just think she's amazing. I hope she's not looking at me
       thinking, "Mom, are the terrible thirties coming on with
       you?"

BB: Can you talk about your workout routine post-baby?
       What does running these marathons do for you?

KH: The running was a great way to get in shape, plus it feels
       so good. My dad and brother had won a marathon and I
       thought this would be a wonderful challenge for me.
       That's the key to working out after the baby. You have
       limited time, so you must find something you really do
       enjoy. As for working out, I run and train with light
       weights. It's about feeling good and not being in this race
       to lose weight in five seconds. You just want to feel strong
       for your family.

BB: What was it like to change your style so dramatically
       over the past few years?

KH: I think it's about evolving as a person. The important
       thing is we're all evolving. As for cutting my hair, it was

very easy to cut it all off. As the mother of a little girl, it's just so much easier to have shorter hair.

BB: How do you deal with all the attention on you?

KH: There is a lot of attention. A lot of attention. I'm aware of what is out there, of course. You know, I married the biggest movie star ever. The attention came with the territory. But it's fine.

BB: Do you want to have more children?

KH: I'd love to have more children. I can bring my mom out to help.

BB: As a mom, how, do you find time to spend with your husband? Any secrets?

KH: You just make the time. Tom has quite a bike collection. It scares me to death and I love it. It's great as long as I don't have to drive.

BB: What is the average day like with Suri?

KH: She's twenty months and we do the normal things. We go to the park. When we were in Berlin there were these beautiful parks. Of course, the paparazzi is just as crazy. There was a lot of attention. But I was impressed with their playgrounds. It's amazing what you become aware of as a mother. You think, "Nice wood on that swing set."

BB: What is it about being a mom that surprised you?

KH: There are a lot of things you just don't know until you're a mom yourself. It's an incredible experience, and you feel a great deal of responsibility and a great deal of love that you never experienced before. It's also even more magical than you envision because how could you envision such joy until it happens?

A-LIST MOM: JENNY McCARTHY

We can't say enough about Jenny McCarthy, mother of Evan, autism advocate, and a mom so nice that she personally writes to other moms to help and inspire them with their care of their autistic children.

Jenny is also a comic actress, so when we asked her to divulge her favorite new mom tip, she said, "Ladies, you gotta, gotta, gotta ask for help. A lot of times you don't want to ask for help, but do it. I know you don't want to be separated from your new child for a second. But at least have someone come over while you take a bath.

"Plan to do one little thing for yourself every single day," she advises. "Believe me, I just wanted to live in my bedroom with Evan and sell Avon products from my home after he was born. He was everything to me, and I didn't want to leave him for a minute. But then I noticed that I was starting to grow armpit hair down to the floor.

"Ladies, armpit hair down to the floor is not attractive to anyone, but least of all yourself. You will not feel good about yourself with armpit hair down to the floor. Stop the madness. When I noticed I could braid that hair I finally asked my mom to come over and help so I could have a nice bath and a shave."

"Evan is amazing. We're so blessed," she says. "He's in school, a typical kid. He's really, really healthy. When I got the news of autism, I said, 'This is what I'm here to do,'" she says. "Anything else, workwise, isn't as much for me. I'm supposed to be doing this with Evan while I'm here. This is my mission."

She also has a great time at home with Evan and her main man, Jim Carrey. "Jim pulls out the glove from *Liar Liar* and chases Evan around the house. They have such a boy-boy relationship. And they run past me with Evan screaming, 'The claw! The claw!'"

THE OTHER GREAT KATE

Ask Kate Beckinsale, the gorgeous Brit and star of *Click*, for parenting advice and she says, "I don't think you can trust advice. Just blast a trail for yourself. I do tell new parents to get some sleep whenever possible or for women to take a nice bath once a day. Treat yourself to that time. I tell men that if your wife is crying a lot and taking care of the baby with no sleep, just buy her some jewelry."

BB EXPERT: ERINN VALENCICH

Forget the generic yellow walls and sad-looking little plastic duck stickers on the walls. We also want you to ban any thoughts of bubble-gum pink paint or boring baby-blue wallpaper. There are nurseries and then there are baby palaces decorated by top Beverly Hills designer and TV show personality Erinn Valencich.

LA-based Erinn is a dynamic young designer whose boutique company, Omniarte Design, transcends its launching point of interior design and is moving steadily toward her goal of an all-embracing lifestyle brand. In just two short years, she has carved out a growing niche: designing homes and events for a youthful, stylish clientele that includes stars like Emmy-winning actress Jaime Pressly, Antonio Sabato Jr., and Jennifer Love Hewitt, and designing the Extra! VIP lounge at Le Meridien hotel in Beverly Hills for the 2006 Academy Awards. "A lot of my clients are people in their twenties and thirties who want an elegant, chic home with a fresh and flexible point of view," she explains.

She's also developing a line of home accessories, including holiday decorations, vases, and candles, adding pillows, bed linens, and, ultimately, furniture, as the line progresses.

The veteran of numerous television appearances on HGTV, *The View*, *Entertainment Tonight*, and *Access Hollywood*, Valencich is also working with a producer to create a series for cable about design and home entertaining. Her TV special *Decked for the Holidays* aired on HGTV, and it will be followed by *Decorating Cents*, *Light It Up!*, and *Fantasy Wedding in a Week*, all airing on HGTV. She is also a Topic Expert on eHow.com, showcasing her ideas to more than one million visitors a day.

She recently completed a nursery for *My Name Is Earl* star Jaime Pressly, whose son, Desi, is really enjoying his new and very cool digs.

We sat down with Erinn to find out how to make your baby's new abode something out of *Better Babies and Gardens*. P.S.: You can find Erinn at ErrinV.com.

BB: Can you tell us a little bit about your celebrity nursery work? What are the current trends when it comes to a swanky 90210 nursery?

EV: I've done many, many nurseries, and some of the people like to keep it private. I can tell you I just did Jaime Pressly's nursery for her son, which was a great experience. I've found that the current trend is that Hollywood celebrities want their nurseries to be more sophisticated and not so babyish. It can still be pink and blue, but the key for anyone—celebrity or nonceleb—is to think about how the room will grow with your child. You don't want to redecorate in two years when all of you are over *Barney*.

BB: How do you get this sophisticated look in a baby nursery?

EV: First, it helps to think about interesting color schemes. I recently did a nursery in chocolate brown and fuchsia. It was very girly but hip at the same time. One of the secrets to a sophisticated nursery is to find adult fabric that has an interesting color palette. I'll buy a yard or two of great fabric for a nursery and use it to make the drapes or pillows. This more adult fabric beautifully counterbalances the sweetness of a baby's room and instantly makes it look more sophisticated. Recently I found a wonderful paisley pattern that could have worked wonderfully in a dining room. I bought a few yards of it and then found an inexpensive matching solid color linen fabric to balance it out. It gave you that perfect baby room look but with a different, more pulled-together feeling.

BB: Where do you look online for great nursery gear for your clients?

EV: This is the day and age of online shopping. One of my favorite sites is modernnursery.com. It's the best because you can outfit your entire nursery from furniture to the bedding. They've got killer things on that site.

Black Book Extra: Modernnursery.com features Oeuf cribs, Bloom highchairs, NurseryWorks cribs, Fleurville diaper bags, and notNeutral nursery-kids furniture. We absolutely adore the ultra-hip and modern Bloombaby White Fresco Loft Highchair for $500. There are also fabulous organic sheets for the newest ones and an amazing selection of really different toys.

BB: Do you have a few calming words for those parents-to-be who are looking at a little room with four white walls thinking, "Where do I start creating my dream nursery?"

EV: Sure! First, this is a happy time, and you should have fun decorating the nursery. I'd start with picking a color palette or a theme if that's what you want. For Jaime we had a jungle theme from *The Jungle Book*. Our colors were sky blue, green, and white. It was very classic and very fresh. And, Jaimie loved that this *Jungle Book* room would last a few years and grow with him. Themes are important, and if you want a ballerina theme for your little girl, that will work. But then pick a color palette that will make the entire nursery look pulled together, and will make shopping easier. Your colors will limit you, which is good because it's actually better if you don't have a thousand options. For that ballerina room I might not do pink but a stunning combination of lavender and gray. Those colors are gorgeous for a little girl's room and will also keep the choices limited.

BB: Are the standard colors of pink, blue, and the all-so-generic yellow really out these days? Or can standards also work if you're a traditional type?

EV: The important thing to know is you don't *have* to do pink, blue, or yellow. You can do a different color palette, but I suggest you keep it light and fun. You can do darker colors, such as a dark purple with lavender and maybe some polka dots or stripes on the walls or in the painting. You can outline purple pillows with pom-pom fringes to make it fun and young. I'm seeing a lot of purple and eggplant in home decorating these days, and it's also coming into the nursery as lavender with soft gray and white accents. It makes a gorgeous girl's room. I also love yellow with light gray for a boy's room. Yellow is actually a hot trend color again, too.

BB: What should you look for when it comes to the baby furniture?

EV: It helps to begin by buying one or two of the basics. Start with a changing table. A lot of people do a dresser with a changing table on top of it. It makes sense; that way you can get rid of the change top later on and use it just as a dresser. You don't want to have to buy new furniture a year or two later. There are even cribs now that turn into beds for children. They just make your life so much easier. I also like vintage pieces like an older dresser mixed with a brand-new crib. You can paint everything the same color white to make it look good and pulled together. I like to go to Craigslist to find vintage. There is also BowerDesigns .com. Their baby furniture is always affordable and they have cute small dressers and beautiful little chairs that look like French antiques. BallardDesigns.com has great wall art to add to the mix.

BB: How do you choose the perfect crib?

EV: I like having a crib that's clean and contemporary. I also like the sleigh cribs. Again, I love the cribs that transition into beds. We found something ideal for Jaime at Pottery Barn. You can take a plain crib and use drapery or netting above it and add a cool mobile. That's a great look.

BB: How can you add a warm, homemade touch to a pulled-together nursery?

EV: A lot of people make their own cool mobiles. If you have a grandmother who knits, ask her to make the animals and you buy the hardware. You can have different mothers and grandmothers make elements for the mobile and change them out. It's a lot more fun than making another baby blanket.

BB: Twins are all the rage in Hollywood. Any advice for parents decorating a room for two?

EV: I'm actually redoing a twin nursery for a couple who have two daughters—Lily and Rose. The girls are two now, and we're doing daybeds on opposite sides of the room. It's very symmetrical. And it's important that the girls have their own daybeds and own areas in their room.

BB: Do some of the rich and famous go way, way, way over the top when decorating for baby? We've heard of couples who spend upward of $200,000 to fill the nursery.

EV: There are people who go way, way over the top. If you feel like it's getting to be too much, then you should scale it back a little bit. Perhaps that ornate drapery is too much. A little pattern and color can make the room stand out. I saw someone do two types of wallpaper, plus ruffles and fringe drapery. I like it better with clean rings and simple drapes. Less can be more.

BB: Many moms have those functional but not so good-looking rocking chairs. Is there any way to find a really great one that doesn't cost a fortune?

EV: I found a modern club chair that was turned into a rocker. It was molded plastic on rocker legs—just adorable. You do want one pop modern piece in the nursery to just mix things up. I did a modern nursery with a rocker that was in pink ultra-suede like a gigantic armchair. They also do a great Mommy and Me rocker set at modernnursery .com. It's super-cute. You can get both rockers in the same color or complimentary ones.

BB: Let's say someone's latest pilot wasn't picked up. How do you have a great nursery on a tight budget?

EV: If you're on a budget, print out photos—black and white ones and oversized ones. Mount them on a white matte with a white frame. Do six or nine on a wall and hang them low—three above, three in the middle, three below. I had someone do this with photos of the future mother's own mother when she was a girl and her father when he was a boy. Then there was a row of the husband's parents when they were little children and even pictures of the great-grandmother as a little girl, plus baby photos of another sibling. It's really fun and cheap. So start looking for those vintage photos of your own mom.

BB: What about the trend of calling an artist and doing a complex animal-themed mural on the walls and white poofy clouds on the ceiling? It seems very common these days, but maybe it's too common.

EV: I think murals are kind of outdated. You can do some subtle clouds on the ceiling, which can be cute. If you really want a mural effect, I'd do art panels. This means you don't paint on the wall but on large panels, which can be removed or moved if you ever buy a new house. For Jaime we did three art panels with *Jungle Book* characters on them. It's like a trip ticket because you can remove the panels or move them around. If she ever gets over them she can get rid of them. Jaime also knew she was going to move and didn't want to invest in a mural and then leave. We did them twenty-four inches by six feet high. And we did take them to the new house. I like the idea of not being stuck with something in a nursery.

BB: Any other great ideas for the baby's walls?

EV: I love vintage wallpaper animals that are actually cut-outs. There is a site called rompstore.com that has vintage giraffes, lions, monkeys, and an almost life-sized tree. The tree base is chocolate, and you pick the colors of the leaves. Everyone loves it! It's a wallpaper tree. They come cut out of the wallpaper and you just put them up, which is very easy. Another tip for walls is really thinking about color. If you're going to do pink, do a super, super-light icy pink, which is almost white, but it's also pink. I just did a little girl's room in icy pink, teal, and cream. The little girl wanted a pink room, but we didn't do the typical pink. The result was a pink so icy and soft that the room actually glows. Then we added cream drapery with teal cherry blooms on them. Again, it's cute but sophisticated. We're doing a khaki and teal headboard, plus a cute crystal chandelier. This room has all the girly elements, and she can grow up in that room and still be cool at age twelve.

BB: We love the idea of chandeliers in the baby's room, and so do the celebs.

EV: I'm doing chandeliers instead of lamp tables all the time. It's also functional because the kids can't knock them over.

BB: And what's a famed parent to do about all those toys that eventually will be strewn across the nursery?

EV: There are lot of different ways you can tackle that, and one thing I've done is a row of shelves low to the ground—child level—so even a toddler can put all of his or her stuffed animals on the shelves. You can still display sentimental toys or even group them. I also love the idea of a settee or a fun bench where the child puts toys to rest. It makes it easy at the end of the day for the kids to clean up and it keeps things organized. If you keep it easy for the kids, then they will group the toys.

A-LIST MOMMY: MARIE OSMOND

She's a little bit country, and a little bit exhausted with eight children to raise as a single mom.

We bow to Marie Osmond, who knows the joys of motherhood. Her secret: "I heard an interesting statement that the best parenting tip is listening. I think that's the most important thing as a mother. You really must stop and truly listen to your child. Put down the cell phone. Stop thinking about work and really hear what your child is saying."

Marie has other great advice for harried moms: "Every time you critique a child, you should have ten positive affirmations for every one criticism. That's my rule," she says.

As a recently divorced mom of eight, doll designer, and contestant on *Dancing with the Stars*, Marie is also developing her own talk show. The secret to being this busy is simple for the Utah native and child star who hit the big-time with her brother Donnie Osmond. "I actually just got off the phone with a friend of mine who is a single mom. We were talking about the fact that 70 percent of our homes in the United States are now single-parent homes.

"That's one of the reasons I'm doing my show. I really want

it to be a destination for busy mothers to take an hour out of their day and make it worth it.

"I think the most important thing for single moms and all women—and this is critical—is to fill your own well because you cannot serve from an empty well," Marie says.

"I'm not talking selfishness, because I don't believe in it. But I do believe in self-love, and I think it's crucial to have that—you know, where it says let Mama stand still and let it all spin around.

"And it's that stillness. It's those quiet moments. I try to find at least a half hour a day where I can just sit and really—you know, whether it's walking or whatever it is, reading—where I can just take that time for me, because it really helps," she says.

Marie looks lean and lovely these days. "Well, of course, I'm working out and I feel good. I got to that place where I was taking care of my parents and my kids, and I put on about five pounds every year for over eight years. Now I have forty pounds off and I feel fantastic. I feel younger than ever. I just did something with the American Heart Association because my mom died of heart disease. My grandmother died of it and my dad suffered from it, too. Since it runs in the family, my son said, "Mom, I need you to lose some weight because we want you to be around.'" She adds, "Being on *Dancing with the Stars* was a great excuse to lose weight. I think it gave women the courage to lose weight. I've gotten some fantastic e-mails, thousands of them, from women saying they're now taking up dancing. This proves life doesn't end at forty."

A-LIST MOMMY: ANGELA BASSETT

Angela Bassett is still waiting to exhale.

On an insane Friday morning at her home outside of Los Angeles, there is no time to even take a deep breath.

It's moving day and the movie star is trying to balance her one-and-half-year-old twins on both hips while giving the moving men some friendly directives.

"That crystal lamp will definitely go with me in the car," she says with a laugh. "I can already see pieces of crystal everywhere in the moving van!"

Talk about multitasking. By the way, she can also do an interview during this chaos.

Bassett, forty-nine, just chuckles when pondering how she does it all . . . and then some.

"Well, the motherhood part is the most challenging," she insists.

Bassett and her husband, actor Courtney Vance, are the parents of twins, Bronwyn Golden and Slater Josiah, born on January 27, 2006, in California through a surrogate.

"A friend of mine is delivering in June and she said, 'Angela, give me some advice, please!'"

"I say to all new mothers, 'You just have to realize now that your babies are smarter than you think they are. They come here brilliant. All they do every single day is learn more. So don't look at these little bitty bundles as if they don't know.'

"They're born a step ahead of Mom and Dad," she insists. "That means you always have to be one step ahead of them and always set high expectations, even if they're just two months old. I would tell my twins, 'You can hold your head up. I know you can hold that bottle. I pray you can sleep through the night.'

"Then I would say, 'Yes, we can. Yes, we can!'" she says.

All that positive thinking sounds good, but at three in the morning it has a way of hitting the skids.

"My girl is a dream, but the boy still wakes up in the middle of the night. I'll go to him and he will put the claws on, which means he grabs me with both hands and both feet while screaming, 'Mommy, Mommy!' Yeah, he works me," says the woman who has been steely tough while handling Ike Turner and Malcolm X on the big screen.

"My husband, Courtney, came home the other day and our son was in the bed with me," she confesses. "We have a deal that the kids aren't supposed to be in our bed.

"Courtney said, 'What is that double breathing I hear in our bed? No monkeys in the bed!'" Bassett says. "I said, 'Honey, he worked me! Yes, he can. Yes, he can!'"

Angela finds inspiration from her own wonderful mom, who was a single mother and a social worker who raised her daughters during tough times in the projects.

"We certainly didn't have it easy," she says. "My mother raised two children on public assistance. My mom taught me during the toughest of times that you just must keep your faith. She set high standards for us, including high moral standards.

"She told us that even in the bleakest financial times that there was one given. My mom would say, 'Truth and love are available for everybody, and they don't cost a dime,'" she recalls. "Mom said, 'Truth and love are not just for the rich or high toned. So whatever you do, just find the truth, love, and justice in this world.'"

She has all the love in the world for twins.

"It's interesting having two. She's sweet; he's rough," she says. "They're not clones.

"Courtney's mom came to visit, and she thought the babies couldn't do certain things. But we don't do everything for them. We want to give them independence. I love the line that parenthood is the only job where if you're good at it then you work yourself out of a job."

How does she do it all?

"With a nanny and a great, capable husband," she says, laughing. "I do find time for myself. My husband can do everything for the babies except braid hair. But he is willing to learn!"

REMOTE PATROL

Even if your parents are running the network and your last name is Zucker, it's time to disconnect the tube from junior's bedroom suite. Yes, take the TV out of your mini mogul's bedroom. Black Book found out that half the kids in America and most in Beverly Hills have a TV in their bedrooms, and the boob tube needs to move out of that space. It's not a great thing for junior to have a TV in his bedroom or her dig: Dr. Leonard Epstein, a professor of pediatrics at State University of New York at Buffalo, found in a study of young children that having that TV in the bedroom meant nine more hours of TV time each week. It gets even worse—70 percent of children who have a TV in their bedroom scored lower grades in math, reading, and language tests. Kids who had video games and computers in their room but no TV got better grades. And kids with those TVs in the bedroom are more likely to be overweight because they sneak snacks like chips and candy bars in to eat while they watch their shows. In fact, the kids with the sets had grades that were lower than kids with no TV in their rooms. Researchers conclude that the TV is a distraction while doing homework, which is then done in a haphazard way between shows. What can parents do to help wean their wee ones off the set? Even if you cut your child's TV time by twenty minutes a day it will help with losing weight and assist in doing better in school.

A-LIST MOMMY: AMY BRENNEMAN

Someone is still always judging Amy.

Amy Brenneman, who is married to director Brad Silberling and has two children, Charlotte Tucker, six, and Bodhi, two, is hiding out in her own driveway. "I just got home and I'm crouching around the side of my house so I can do this interview and my children don't see me," says the star of the TV hit *Judging Amy*. It's hard to be a working mom, and Brenneman is working in key roles these days. She just starred in the action film *88 Minutes* opposite Al Pacino and on the TV series *Private Practice*, the *Grey's Anatomy* spinoff.

We asked for her best mom tip, and Brenneman didn't hesitate: "I just get down on the floor with them. That's always the answer to a lot of things. If things feel discombobulated in the house—and face it, we all live hectic lives, between school and driving to activities—I'll just lie down on the floor and let them flop on me. You just have to let it rip," she says with a laugh.

CANDY FOR BABES AND BABIES

While doing all this writing about pregnancy and cravings, your Black Book gals decided to take a break and head over the pond to check out our favorite Scottish and British products and gift stores. Plus, we just wanted to eat some really good Cadbury milk chocolates. During our baby binge, we found out about a wonderful British baby secret the Americans haven't caught onto . . . until now. (Well, probably except for Gwyneth and Madonna.)

English mums like Sharon Osbourne and her rocker hubby pick up Farley's Rusks for their friends who are having babies. These are British treats for little ones, and have been used for more than 120 years. They are a specially designed snack for babies and toddlers (starting at four months), enriched with vitamins and minerals essential for healthy growth and development. It's the perfect food to wean through to toddler years. There are many ways of serving this unique food to your baby—like crushing the rusks in a clean bowl and adding some baby's milk or boiled water. Rusks can also be crushed up and mixed with fruit or vegetable purée or as a tasty low-sugar dessert by adding yogurt or custard. They're a great finger food and in-between meal snack filled with iron, calcium, and prebiotics but no genetically modified ingredients, which are allowed here in the United States in baby foods. Farley's Rusks are available at OH Fancy That British Gifts in Tarzana, California, for five dollars or online at ohfancythat@sbcglobal.net.

My son had to draw his family for a school project. Then he had to tell his teacher about the picture, which included all of the family and the dog. Joaquin told his teacher, "Here is my daddy. My daddy is nice. I'm nice to him. Here is my sister. She is nice. She always lets me play games with her. This is Michael. He's always nice. This is my dog. The dog is nice. And there's Mommy. She's coming back from the Hamptons. She is going to take me to Disneyland." Excuse me. I'm not nice. I'm the only one who is not nice. He told her everyone was nice, including the dog. What about Mommy!

—**Kelly Ripa**

HELLO HELENA

Don't tell Helena Bonham Carter what to do with her pregnancy. Carter, who was eight months expecting with her and Tim Burton's baby, told us, "People—particularly men—say with surprise, 'You're still drinking caffeine?' as if I'm performing a criminal act on my unborn as I tuck into my treasured one-a-day cup of tea or coffee. Yeah. You try nine months of gestation before you start censoring my diet. Your mother was probably on vodka, and do you have three heads?"

BB EXPERT: LESLIE LEHR

Leslie Lehr is a mother, prize-winning author, screenwriter, and essayist. Her books include the novel *66 Laps*, the humorous parenting books *Welcome to Club Mom* and *The Happy Helpful Grandma Guide* (now excerpted on FisherPrice.com), and the celebrity design book *Wendy Bellissimo: Nesting* (featured on *Oprah*). Her film *Heartless* was a romantic thriller, and she's currently working on a mother-daughter story of obsession called *The Long Way Home*.

For *Mommy Wars*, the controversial book about the battle between working moms and stay-at-home moms, Leslie (who considers herself a working-at-home mom) contributed the essay "I Hate Everybody." Motherhood also inspired her essay in *The Honeymoon's Over*, called "Welcome to the Club"—about how she resisted being a statistic to avoid having her kids grow up in a "broken" home. When she realized being a good role model was more important for her kids, she began celebrating her second act and wrote the popular novel *Wife Goes On*, a heartwarming and hilarious story of four women, three of them moms, who help each other live happier ever after.

Leslie gave Black Book some insight on parenting after divorce. Check out the rest of her work at leslielehr.com and wife-goes-on.com.

BB: What kind of perspective do you have on motherhood?

LL: Being a new mom is what lead me to be a writer in the first place. As an educated career woman, I read everything I could get my hands on and thought I was prepared. *Ha!* The change was so radical that I started venting at two in the morning in short essays—poignant, upbeat essays, but really a cry from the heart. They evolved into my first book, *Welcome to Club Mom: The*

End of Life as You Know It. But the publisher thought the subtitle was too negative, so they changed it to *Welcome to Club Mom: The Adventure Begins.* And there's no denying the adventure of 24/7 responsibility. I nursed my next child through fifty-three phone interviews for my second book to keep her quiet. Even now motherhood trumps career. During a recent National Public Radio interview for *Wife Goes On*, while the host read my credits to introduce me live on the air, my kids were pounding on my office door whining about dinner. At least my nipples didn't get sore this time.

BB: Is there really a "Club Mom" mind-set? Give us a few examples.

LL: Oh, yes. I recently had lunch with an old friend, an executive who has no kids, and at first I had no idea what to talk about. I was afraid if I whipped out their picture or even mentioned what they were up to, it would be either bragging or boo-hoo-ing. A week later, as the only writer at a luncheon for the Women's Leadership Council of Los Angeles, a group of high-powered law partners and CEOs, I was never at a loss for conversation because we had so much in common as mothers. It's the same wherever I go. Seriously, who else knows the pain of a bleary-eyed woman cruising the diaper aisle at dawn?

BB: What was your biggest feel-good secret during your pregnancy?

LL: Massages. I found a guy who had a trampoline bed massage table. *Heaven!* It's also the only time you can demand foot rubs. And ditch the restroom line.

BB: What was your biggest beauty secret during your pregnancy?

LL: Accessories, the bigger the better—scarves, earrings, everything to scale off my belly. This included my hair, which grew down to my pleasantly plump bottom. I took advantage of all that hormonal hair growth to the full Madonna effect. It feels very sexy, which is a huge plus after hearing the baby's father tell his friends it's like sleeping with a pony keg.

BB: How did you lose the weight after giving birth?

LL: I figured it took nine months to get that weight and I'd give it nine months to get rid of it—especially when nursing. Using the stroller was my favorite way to exercise. That was all about meeting moms and their strollers at every corner—like a parade. Mommy and Me classes are great, too. It's the only place you can admit to mind-numbing boredom before bath time.

BB: How is being a mother who is divorced different from being a mother who is married?

LL: Depends on the mom. My mom was busy working and studying for her PhD when I was growing up, so I think I overcompensated by smothering my kids with attention. When I divorced and had to spend more time at business meetings and, finally, dating, they were mighty relieved to get rid of me. My ex-husband traveled so much that I used to be jealous of divorced women who had every other weekend off. Now that I'm divorced I still don't have any weekends off but there sure is a lot less laundry. Since I have girls, we're a closer unit. Not like girlfriends—I'm still the mom—but we can shop without rushing home to deal with dinner.

BB: What is the best piece of advice you received about pregnancy/mothering and about being a divorced mom?

LL: When you're pregnant, go out as much as possible, but know where the bathrooms are. When you're a mom, asking for help is not weak; it's smart. When you are divorced, be sure to carve out time for yourself. In fact, do that always.

BB: What is the best piece of advice you can give to someone else about pregnancy/mothering and being a divorced mom?

LL: There is no such thing as Having It All—at least not at the same time.

BB: What is the absolute biggest, fattest lie about pregnancy or motherhood that is perpetuated and should be exposed?

LL: That you don't poop during childbirth. You do. It's gross, but there you have it. Also, the whole process is a heck of a lot more messy than you can imagine.

BB: How do you feel about the pressure new moms seem to have nowadays, thanks to Hollywood, to look perfect, lose all the baby weight in three seconds, and get back to work five minutes after having a child?

LL: Think airbrushing. Also think personal trainers, nutritionists, chefs, hairdressers, and wardrobe stylists. And think of all the swear words you can. Then blurt them out and blame it on hormones.

BB: What is the funniest story you could tell us about being a first-time mother?

LL: I can describe the day from hell, which is not unlike many other days that all blur together. My dad is a scientist and wanna-be movie star who was an extra in every film I worked on before the baby was born. So he was disappointed when I couldn't drag my newborn on location with me and passed on a movie in Prague. He called on my birthday, one of those holidays that disappear when life no longer revolves around you. I hadn't slept at all. My baby was colicky all night, so I alternated between laundry and dishes and feeding and diapers and bills and rocking and crying—me crying—and that's when the phone rang. So my dad chats cheerily about his latest lecture as I'm trying to cradle the phone on my shoulder and burp the baby, who spits up on me then suddenly reeks to high heaven. That's when my dad wishes me a happy birthday and asks me when I plan to go back to work.

I didn't argue about his definition of work; I was missing the money part, too, but I didn't have any plan past the diaper table—and now the doorbell was ringing and the dryer was buzzing and the baby was tearing out a strand of my hair. I sighed and told my dad I had no idea. He was seriously perplexed. "A smart girl like you," he mused. "But what do you do all day?" I looked around the decimated kitchen and thought about all I'd done in the last few hours and said, "I could write a book." So I did.

BB: What is the BEST part about being a mother who went through a divorce, survived it, and thrived and is also a successful author and essayist?

LL: Every day I wake up feeling happy. Okay, not stupid happy, but happy with who I am. I know who that is now, and it makes me feel powerful. I made a lot of choices in my life, some good, some bad, some by default, but I'm in charge now—and this is it! I look in the mirror and see the person I want to be—with the potential to be even more. I'm grateful to have a voice through my writing, and that I can share that with other women. Maybe I can make a difference.

I think we learn more by picking ourselves up after disappointments and, while I hope my daughters skip the hard parts, I have to believe they will know how to bounce back and move on. I hope they have learned how to be treated, how to choose the right kind of man, and, most important, how to make their own dreams come true.

I'm excited for them to begin their own journeys. Not only so they stop stealing my clothes, but also because I'm excited about their prospects. Certainly they will know that no matter what, I am always here for them. Now that they're teenagers people ask if I'm sad about the prospect of an empty nest. That couldn't be further from the truth. Sure, I get teary just thinking about it, but I've devoted my life to help my children become happy and productive adults. I didn't know I was capable of such love, but I know that they are. They may have false starts or take paths that surprise me, but the rest is up to them. Life is a gift with no strings attached. Who knows what they will accomplish? I feel proud already.

CHAPTER 6

How to Have a Baby and an A-list Life!

She doesn't look like a mom. She looks like a babysitter.
—**Kelly Ripa, on the highest compliment her children can give another woman**

HOW TO PLAN A BABYMOON

A-list couples need to take one last romantic getaway before their lives are changed forever. In Hollywood it's called a babymoon. But you don't want to go to a place where he will scuba and you will sit alone at the pool.

How can you plan the perfect babymoon? First you need to make sure that travel time is minimized (no ten-hour layovers), there are good medical facilities nearby, and the activities are good (pregnancy massages, anyone?). Rule out cruises (many won't let pregnant women on after twenty-four to twenty-seven weeks).

Black Book has learned of three super-hot destinations:

- The Plantation Inn in Charleston, South Carolina: Romantic, luxurious, old hotel with gorgeous rooms, and

the town has a great walking tour. The hotel even provides ice cream at night, a baby-care package, and prenatal massages.

- Half Moon Bay in Jamaica: Beautiful beaches for R&R
  and great virgin piña coladas, plus foot massages and a
  welcome baby onesie.

- Peter's Island in the British Virgin Islands: Picnic on the
  beach, with sparkling apple juice for you and champagne
  for him. They will also bring in a child-care education
  expert to teach you baby prep!

YOUR KIDS ARE WHAT YOU EAT!

Want your kids to love veggies? Eat them while pregnant
and while breast-feeding and you won't struggle as hard to get
your kids to eat healthy later on. In a study at the Monell Chemical Senses Center, a research institute in Philadelphia, researchers have found that this is a way of "indoctrinating"
your child's taste buds, and you can even get them to like spe-
cific veggies like broccoli, Brussels sprouts, cabbage, or green
beans by eating them before your child is born. Flavors from a
mom-to-be's diet are transmitted through amniotic fluid and
mother's milk. The study proves that babies learn to develop
tastes for foods that their mother eats before they are born.
During the study, pregnant and nursing moms drank carrot
juice, and their kids loved and craved carrots much more than
the moms who avoided carrot juice. It also works for fruits.
Also interesting is that when breast-feeding moms started to
eat green beans a few times a week, babies who originally
shunned green beans suddenly did a turn-around and loved

them. By the way, it's not your child's fault if he or she hates veggies. Kids hate anything that tastes even a bit bitter. So if you tweak their taste buds, it will help them crave the good stuff later on.

LISTEN UP

What is pink noise? It's the hottest thing with A-list celebs in Hollywood like Julia and Reese, who put their babies to sleep with this creative, full-length, full-spectrum noise designed to recreate the sounds in the womb. Scientific research shows that pink noise is actually a very effective sound to soothe a newborn. Check it out at www.thewhitenoisealbum.com /pinknoise.html.

FINALLY! AN ALCOHOL-FREE, NATURAL HAND SANITIZER!

If you're anything like us harried Black Book mums, you have a bottle of Purell in your It Bag (the horror if it leaks on the Gucci), in your car, on your counter, next to your changing table, and on the list of things requested weekly by your child's preschool teacher. (Don't you love all the gummy, half-smeared lists around the house? We even imagine Jessica has a list somewhere that says: Buy diapers, make out with Cash . . .)

But we digress.

If you're like us, you also hate how that icky hand sanitizer smells and how it stings, and you're not sure if you should actually use it on your toddler, even though he put his hands in the toilet . . . at the mall. (Insert your own shriek here.)

Turns out we have good reason to be concerned about our

kids using some name-brand sanitizers, since many are 62 percent ethyl alcohol. Uh, hello . . . that's flammable, toxic, and dries the heck out of human skin. Think of all those poor kids with their cracked winter hands crying whenever their mean mommy forces them to use the sanitizer, but it's a necessity when you run into a neighbor at the store who tells you about their kid's nasty strep throat at the exact moment said infected kid is licking your child's arm for no reason other than trying to deny you the chance to go the Emmys with a clear head and not visions of a 102-degree fever.

Thankfully, after eight long years in the laboratory, the good folks at CleanWell have just released the first natural hand sanitizer. Made entirely of botanical extracts, CleanWell hand sanitizers kill 99.9 percent of germs—even the really bad ones like E. coli, salmonella, and staph—yet actually restore your skin, leaving it soft and sweet-smelling, thanks to aloe vera and natural citrus essence. It's all-natural, hypoallergenic, and completely kid safe—so safe they aren't even required to post warnings on the label. Of course, it's for external use only, so don't let your kid drink it, but it's far better than my old hand sanitizer, which cautions to "keep out of reach from children."

CleanWell is chemical free right down to the harvesting of their natural products, which are grown without pesticides or fertilizers. The active germ-fighting ingredient in CleanWell is Ingenium, which is harnessed from thyme and other essential oils.

CleanWell is available in a spray bottle and as wipes. Our kids are in love with it, and so are we. You can find it at Target and Whole Foods, and online at cleanwelltoday.com.

MOMS GIVE US A LINE

We all know that everyone is going green these days, and most moms want to be the first in their hood to show they are environmentally aware. Here's the hottest trend in Hollywood, and it won't cost much to get you in the pack. Just go back to the 1950s and grab a clothesline. Yes, old-fashioned backyard clotheslines, like we used to see in the movies, that the moms would talk over to their neighbor each morning as they were hanging out the family's freshly washed clothes to dry in the soft spring and summer breeze. Stars like Rachel Bilson and Matthew Rhys are all "lining up" to get their clothesline for the outdoors. The celebs feel that installing retractable outdoor poles on the sides of their homes rather than using electric dryers is their way of going green and conserving energy.

SUSAN'S GOT US SUSSED

Susan Sarandon is the type of super-mom who is so cool that you want her to hold seminars to share her mom secrets. Luckily Black Book caught up with her in Long Beach, California, during the Grand Prix races to talk all things parental. With her red hair flowing and wearing a floral long jacket, Sarandon might look like a movie star, but she sounds like any other mom on the planet. "My whole life I tried not to work too much during the school year and carted my kids around. Now they're older and they say, 'Mom, please leave. Go. Immediately,'" she says with a warm laugh. "I have two out of the house now and I practically have to work with my daughter Eva just to spend time with her."

Hmmmm . . . how did she get the name Eva (pronounced ev-ah)? "I joke with her that her name is so special that the Beatles wrote a song for her. When she was a little girl, I used to sing, 'Strawberry Fields for Eva.'"

Black Book asked Susan for her best parenting tip, and she confided, "Learn how to apologize to your kids."

Excuse us? "No, it's really important to learn how to say

you're sorry to your children because there will be times when you are sorry," she says. "Your kids need to learn that mistakes happen in life and you need to get over it, say you're sorry, and get on to the next spot.

"I think it's also really important for mothers to learn how to forgive themselves," Susan says. "You need to forgive yourself for not being perfect. You also have to say, 'I want to spend time with my kids so maybe the fridge won't get defrosted, but so what.' What's really important here? Even if you're the world's most perfect mother, that's a burden to your kids."

BB EXPERTS: LIANE WEINTRAUB AND SHANNAN SWANSON

After many years of close friendship and creative collaboration, Liane Weintraub and Shannan Swanson started Tastybaby. Liane describes the first meeting between the two best friends as being "like falling in love," and today they consider each other family as well as business partners who created Tastybaby.

Liane and Shannan tell us: "When we both became mothers, we started making organic food for our babies. We didn't spend much time considering whether we would do that—it just seemed normal not to want to feed jarred, processed food to these incredible beings we'd carried in our bodies and nurtured so carefully and lovingly. Also, we've both been major foodies all our lives—in fact, that's what bonded our friendship in the first place! So after years of cooking together for ourselves, our families, and our friends, it was only natural that we would be cooking for our children.

"We have to be honest: What started out as a purely joyful experience—steaming and puréeing beautiful organic ingredients—soon turned into quite a chore. After being busy with work and commitments all day, the last thing either of us wanted to do was spend our precious time at home bonding with our blenders instead of with our babies . . . but what choice did we have? There were no options on the market for healthy, delicious food that was safe for babies, and the idea of feeding our little ones three-year-old fruits and vegetables that had been sitting in jars was too upsetting for words. So, we rolled up our sleeves and started cooking. That's how Tastybaby was born!

"But we wanted to do more than just start a healthy baby food business—we wanted it to be a force to help make the world a better place. We have both been committed to green practices, and we made sure to find planet-friendly packaging that is biodegradable or recyclable and we print with soy- and vegetable-based inks. We do everything we can to be sensitive to the environment, from sourcing the highest quality ingredients as locally as possible to working with vendors and partners who support important things like sustainable agriculture, Fair Trade, using alternative energy sources, and so forth. We needed Tastybaby to be be a company and a product we would feel good about. After all, since we make food for the next generation, we feel we should try to protect the planet they are going to inherit while we're at it.

"We feel we're on our way to making a difference in the world by offering a wonderful nutritional start for babies and by sending out a clear and consistent message about social responsibility and a new, fun, fashionable approach to green-living on our Web site, Tastybaby.com.

BB: Tell us about Tastybaby, how and why you started the company?

L&S: Now we are officially among the "mom-preneurs" who are helping make life easier, healthier, and more FUN for people like us. We consider that to be a really great honor, and we try to keep in mind every day that our customers are like cherished girlfriends who are putting their trust in us.

BB: Isn't it easier to just run to the grocery store and grab a jar of the old standby baby food to feed our little ones?

L&S: Well, yes, we suppose. And if easier is your only priority, then that's what you should do. But before you make that decision, you should be informed about what you are choosing. In our opinion (as well as in the opinion of most health professionals and nutritionists we've spoken to), jarred foods are never the optimal choice for anyone's diet—especially that of a baby or child. The simple fact is that in order to maintain food in a jar at room temperature and with a long shelf life (often three years!), food must be highly processed. That means it's cooked at a very high temperature for a very long time before it's vacuum-packed into a glass or plastic container with a lid that has a rubber seal on it. There are now jarred baby foods made with organic ingredients, which offer an advantage over non-organic products because they don't contain pesticides, but that doesn't change how these products are processed—by the time the homogenizing and pasteurizing and vacuum-packing is completed, it seems doubtful that many of the vital nutrients are left in the organic ingredients that went into these products.

Our products, which are blast-frozen using state-of-the-art technology, are minimally processed because they are frozen—essentially "suspended in time"—within minutes of cooking. This makes it impossible for unpleasant things such as bacteria, yeasts, and molds to grow, which means our products are as pure and natural as the tiny customers we make them for!

According to the American Cancer Society, "frozen foods can be more nutritious than fresh foods because they are often picked ripe and quickly frozen, whereas fresh foods may loose some of their nutrients in the time between harvesting and consumption."

BB: Why do you think so many celebrities are drawn to Tastybaby?

L&S: We are always pleased when our customers respond positively to our products—it's an incredible thrill to know that you've affected someone in a positive way. Among these "fans" happen to be a lot of celebrities, which is hugely gratifying because most of these people have access to just about anything and everything, so the fact that they've chosen Tastybaby is really flattering. We think celebs love Tastybaby for several different reasons: For one, Hollywood has been a leading force for spreading the word about the importance of organics and green living, so the purity of our products and the integrity of our choices regarding sourcing of ingredients and the materials we use for our packaging really resonate with celebs. Also, because Tastybaby has a true "fashion-forward" look, our design has a lot of eye candy appeal to it—that's why you see celebs like Cindy Crawford, Angie Harmon, and Nia Long carrying our eco-tote bags and wearing our Tasty T-shirts . . . it may sound egotistical, but there's just something fabulous about our brand that attracts not only celebrities but people with great taste and a sense of fun!

BB: It sounds a little odd, but we understand that not only do the children enjoy your food but moms love it as well and it even helps them lose weight after having a baby. Can you tell us about that and how they incorporate it into their own healthy meals?

L&S: We don't think it sounds odd at all! If the thought of incorporating what your baby eats into your own diet seems strange, well, then maybe what you're feeding your baby is the problem. Since our products are simply 100 percent organic foods that have been puréed and frozen, there's actually nothing strange about them. What makes them appropriate for babies (that they're pure and healthy) is precisely what makes them great for everyone else!

We started hearing from moms that when they tasted our food as they were feeding their babies, they found they couldn't stop eating it themselves . . . they told us they were buying "one for baby and one for me," and then their toddlers and older children got intrigued. That's what led us to start developing recipes that incorporate our foods—some are appropriate for babies (adding age-appropriate elements such as cereal to our fruit flavors or pasta to our veggies), others for older kids (like our Sweetie Pie cupcakes), and some are just for adults (like our Life's a Peach Bellinis, which we served at Jessica Alba's baby shower, or the Bango coladas we created for Tori Spelling).

BB: Could you give us a recipe or two incorporating Tastybaby products into standard fare?

L&S: Here's one of our faves for people of any age. Joely Fisher is a huge fan.

Bango Smoothie

4 packs Tastybaby Bangos
1 cup organic apple juice
2 cups low-fat or fat-free vanilla yogurt
1 cup ice cubes
1 ripe banana (optional)

Combine all the ingredients in a blender and blend until smooth. If the smoothie is too thick, thin with a little more apple juice. Pour into 4 large glasses and serve.

And here's a great recipe created by chef Angela Boccuzzi-Gaines for Elisabeth Rohm's baby shower:

Squash 'Em Ravioli with Brown Butter Sage Sauce

8 containers Tastybaby Squash 'Em
¼ teaspoon ground allspice
¼ teaspoon ground nutmeg
1 teaspoon ground cinnamon
¼ cup Parmesan cheese
25 wonton wrappers
1 egg white, lightly beaten
2 tablespoons unsalted butter
2 tablespoons chopped fresh sage leaves
Salt and freshly ground black pepper to taste

1. Fill a deep pot with lightly salted water and bring to a boil.

2. In a large bowl, mix the Squash 'Em with the allspice, nutmeg, cinnamon, and cheese.

3. To make the ravioli, place a wonton wrapper on a clean, flat surface. Brush the edges with the egg white. Place about 1 tablespoon of the Squash 'Em mixture in the middle of the wonton. Cover with a second wonton wrapper. Repeat until all the remaining wonton wrappers and Squash 'Em have been used.

4. Drop a few ravioli at a time into the boiling water and cook for 2 to 4 minutes, until tender. Don't overcrowd the pot. Drain and keep warm until sauce is prepared.

5. To make the sauce, melt the butter in a skillet over medium-low heat. DO NOT BURN THE BUTTER. Stir in the sage. Continue to cook and stir until the sage is crisp but not browned. Season with salt and pepper. Place the raviolis on 4 serving plates and drizzle with the sauce.

BB: What is the favorite item in your Tastybaby line that both the moms and children love?

L&S: Of course everyone's palates are different, including babies, so there are going to be babies (and adults) who simply aren't keen on, say, peaches or peas. But other than allowing for personal taste, we've noticed that everyone loves all our products because they don't taste at all like what people associate with baby food (bland, watery, and flavorless). We've heard stories of "addictions" to Sweetie Pie (in fact, we served it to our families as a side dish for Thanksgiving!) and Peas on Earth (this makes a fantastic base for a quick pea soup). But our overall winner would have to be Life's a Peach, since most people, regardless of their age, simply love the taste of fresh peaches. Life's a Peach is made from pure, organic white peaches (no additives!) that have been simply puréed and blast-frozen to truly capture the sweet taste of summer. When Stella McCartney asked us to host an event for her, we created our now-famous Life's a Peach Bellini in her honor. In case you're wondering, here's how you make it:

Life's a Peach Bellini

1 teaspoon Life's a Peach purée
4 to 6 ounces champagne
1 peach slice

Thaw the Life's a Peach purée and spoon it into a glass. Slowly add the champagne and stir gently. Garnish with a peach slice.

Note: You can also make it in a pitcher by combining 1 to 2 four-ounce servings of Life's a Peach with a bottle of champagne.

BB: Most women are desperate to lose weight after baby. Do you have any suggestions on how to do that with and without your food?

L&S: We've been hearing stories about celebs and others going on the "baby food diet" with Tastybaby. We're not nutritionists, so we couldn't comment on the diets, but we definitely think Tastybaby foods are delicious, low-calorie snacks and great additions to anyone's diet—it's not just for babies!

BB: What was your biggest feel-good secret during your pregnancies?

L&S: It's so important to take care of yourself during pregnancy—not just in the obvious ways with good nutrition, but also mentally and emotionally. Crazy as some of them might be, cravings are just your body's way of telling you what it needs, so we say give in to them—within reason, of course!

BB: What were your biggest beauty secrets during your pregnancies?

S: I really enjoyed prenatal yoga throughout my first pregnancy. The classes were great for relaxation, and I made wonderful friends among the moms-to-be.

L: I made a promise to myself that I would schedule monthly facials while I was pregnant. Whatever was going on south of my neck, at least I had a nice complexion to focus on!

BB: How did you lose the weight after giving birth?

L&S: Well, the truth is that our routines probably weren't ideal. Liane's son was a newborn and Shannan was four months pregnant when we started Tastybaby, so we were working and juggling motherhood, pregnancy, breast-feeding, and everything else at the same time. The bottom line is, there's lots of great advice to be had. For us, we couldn't make time for traditional workouts, so we would just have to work it in whenever we could without detracting from our work or home lives. Sometimes you just have to get creative . . . and give yourself a break!

BB: As busy moms, how do you take care of yourself? Any quick tips for beauty, diet, or exercise as a mom? Any tips you gained from your celebrity customers?

L&S: We'll admit it: Sometimes it's a challenge. It's hard to make the decision to go get a manicure when we need to be working. Then, when we have "free" time, it doesn't feel right to be away from our kids too much. To the best of our abilities, we incorporate our business and our children into every aspect of our lives. The fun thing about having daughters is that they LOVE beauty treatments, and it's a special thing to be able to share with them.

Also, the best thing about having a business partner who's your best friend is that we're on the same page in terms of beauty, diet, and exercise. We eat many meals together and we've been able to inspire each other in terms of eating healthy . . . although we're major foodies and we both love a good gourmet meal! Another great thing is that since we need to spend time talking about our business and brainstorming new ideas, there's no reason this has to be done sitting down! We love taking long beach walks or mountain hikes in Malibu as we plan our next steps and Tastybaby's future. It's good for our bodies and really gets our creative juices flowing.

Our office staff is mostly women, and we've made a pact to support each other. One new thing we've all started is to encourage each other to drink more water during the day. Every time someone refills her glass from the water cooler, we all give a thumbs-up!

BB: What was the one item, food, clothing, or ritual that helped you get through your pregnancy?

L: In terms of clothing, I started wearing Hanro tank tops during my first pregnancy because they are super-soft and they stretched, along with my belly . . . I still wear them almost every day! Foodwise, my husband makes the most amazing shakes. I have no idea what goes into them except that he uses almond milk for the base and then adds all kinds of potions and powders (everything from freeze-dried spirulina to whey protein to who-knows-what) and the end result is something I got hooked on during pregnancy. Now I cannot start my day without one of his shakes!

S: Pregnancy jeans by Earl were my salvation, fashion-wise, and tons of cocoa butter kept stretch marks away! One thing that was fun was that Liane and I had pregnancies that were staggered by a year (my daughter, Louisa, is a year older than her daughter, Ava, and her son, Cole, is a year older than my son, Sonny), so we were able to trade and share pregnancy clothes. Our closets were in constant rotation, and one of us was always borrowing the other one's maternity stuff, while the other one was borrowing nonpregnancy things. And now our kids get each other's hand-me-downs, so the cycle continues. We think of it as our own take on "Reduce, Reuse, Recycle"!

BB: What is the best piece of advice you received about pregnancy and mothering?

L&S: We've gotten some incredible advice from really special people whom we truly admire. We'll share a few with Black Book readers.

Gabrielle Reece

What are the most important ways you keep your family healthy?

By being a healthy example. You can't tell your kids to go outside and play or eat healthy—you have to get outside yourself and teach them how to enjoy healthy food. Children are smart and they will learn intuitively what is good about your day-to-day actions.

Cindy Crawford

What trait do you hope your kids don't inherit?

I hope my kids don't inherit my perfectionism. I work hard at accepting that sometimes it's okay to just be good enough!

Greg Kinnear

What does "family" mean to you?

Being part of something, sharing the good times and the tough times, but sharing . . .

Angie Harmon

What's the "tastiest" thing about your family?

The "tastiest" thing about our family is the giggles. Those girls can giggle and squeal with the best of 'em. Especially when we chase them through the house. . . . It sounds like there are twenty little girls at a Justin Timberlake concert and they're all in the front row! Thank God I have a few years before that happens!!

BB: What was the absolute biggest, worst lie about pregnancy or motherhood that is perpetuated and should be exposed?

L&S: Without a doubt, the biggest lie is that as mothers we can "do it all." As anyone who's spent time on Tastybaby .com knows, we talk a lot about all the different facets of parenthood and the challenges of creating (not to mention maintaining) a balance among all of these. In fact, "balance" is something of a mantra for us—it's even part of our tagline ("The Flavor of a Balanced Life"), and if we were the types to get tattoos (we're not, by the way, mostly because of the PAIN factor!), we'd probably both have that word permanently emblazoned on our bodies—that's how focused we are on trying to achieve the elusive balance between work, motherhood, wifehood, good citizenry, and, to be blunt about it, not letting ourselves go in the process! That said, the idea that you can be all things to all people at all times is an utter lie, and buying into it is a dangerous trap.

BB: How do you feel about the pressure new moms seem to have nowadays—to look perfect, lose the baby weight, and get back to work five minutes after having a child?

L&S: That kind of pressure is really awful and terribly unfair. If there's anything we can accomplish with the message part of our business, it's to help empower women not to succumb to it. On Tastybaby.com we have wonderful insight, expert advice, and first-person blogs from celebrities and regular moms alike who raise important questions and address these questions in ways every woman can relate to. One of our contributors, Shari Sonta, is a working mom who finds the time to blog for us while she's pumping! She put it very well in one of her posts: "I don't care what position *Working Mother* magazine takes—being a full-time working mom in today's corporate culture really, really stinks. I keep hearing rumors of companies that offer flextime, job sharing, and telecommuting options, but I think that's a color picture in the Land of Oz, Inc."

The truth is, no one can pull off the illusion of the

"perfect life," and anyone who seems to is probably giving up something else, so we feel it's very important for women to do what's best for THEMSELVES and their families. Everything in life is a trade-off (even having a business as wonderful as Tastybaby takes us away from our families), so try make your choices count for something!

BB: What are the best parts about being pregnant and a mother?

L&S: We can both honestly say that getting pregnant and becoming moms was the most wonderful, natural, and *necessary* thing that either of us has ever experienced. We can see how it's not something everyone should do in their lives (in spite of a huge amount of pressure on every female to reproduce . . . but that's another topic for another book!), but for both of us it has been what we *needed* to do in our lives. To top it all off, had we not had children we never would have started Tastybaby, and then what would all those adorable babies have to eat?!

UM-BRELLA, ELLA, ELLA

Any given day here in sunny California you can spot a Hollywood mom playing on the beaches of Malibu or Santa Monica with one of her little ones. However, in Tinsel Town the starlets are well aware of just how early skin damage can start, so they take all precautions to ensure that their little love-lies stay looking that way and avoid exposure to the dreaded sun.

This A-list behavior include their choice of beach umbrellas.

The Anna Collection by Beach Pockets is for the elite and most discriminating beach-goers and vacationers. Hollywood moms would never just put sunscreen on their kids for a day at the beach—they bring along their beach umbrella with SPF 50 in the fabric, ensuring double duty that they or their children will not be in the harmful rays.

Stars like Barbara Walters, Tori Spelling, and Ali Laundry are all fans of the new product that was conceived (no pun intended) and designed by a working mom with towheaded children with sun sensitive skin, and who was also frustrated by beach umbrellas that would not stay anchored to the sand.

So not only will Mom be protecting herself and the kids, it's also environmentally friendly because mothers don't have to worry about their flimsy umbrellas blowing away in the wind. The pocket umbrella features three pockets that attach to the lightweight pole barrel and when filled with sand prevent it from blowing away.

Creator Barbara Bigford says, "It is also respectful to the environment because when you are finished with your day you empty the sand from the pockets back onto the beach, pull up your light-weight umbrella and pole, and head to the car. It's easy for Mom to carry, has a built-in sun protection factor of 50 in the material, and stays put with beach sand."

Pamela Anderson, eat your heart out. It sounds better than *Baywatch*.

Prices range from $19.99 to $78.00, and they are available at beachpockets.com and at Wal-Marts in some states.

SCRIBBLE, SCRIBBLE

Your kids are drawn to their bedroom walls. And, oh boy, it shows. The consensus: Crayon squiggly lines do not enhance your faux finish. The solution: Coat the room with Yoyamart's

Chalkboard-Magnetic Paint. Just a few dips into the container will transform their walls into blackboards. Hand over the chalk and let Picassolina create a masterpiece, pretend to teach school, or just scribble. What's more, kiddies can even display artwork by tacking a magnet on top. The magical process defies explanation, so we wouldn't ask how it's done.

The details are, after all, a little sketchy.

A-LIST MOMMY: HELEN HUNT

We can tell you who Helen Hunt is mad about these days. It's her three-year-old daughter, Makena, and her longtime boyfriend. Black Book sat down with the star of *Mad About You* and *As Good as It Gets* to talk about combining motherhood with a frenzied work life.

BB: The character in your latest movie, *Then She Found Me*, longs for a baby and is at that age where she wonders if she will have one. Did you also get to that stage in life?

HH: I wasn't so busy with my career and then remembered to have a baby. The circumstances of my life and my body conspired to make it not the simplest thing in the world. The timing had to happen when it was right. I'm an older mother and I'm more tired than I would have been in my twenties. But I'm also glad my daughter isn't subjected to me at twenty. There is so much more wisdom.

BB: How has your life changed since your daughter was born? Any advice for new moms?

HH: You learn how great it is to have grandparents and friends who are willing to help. I was sent a terrific Broadway play last year and my heart pounded when I read it. I was terrified that I'd really want to do it. But then I thought that missing her bedtime was something I wouldn't ever want to do. I'm not comfortable with not being around. I just can't do it. It makes jumping on a plane to do a job pretty hard to do. As for advice, if you've just had a baby, tell people not to send you presents and instead to make dinner and leave it on the front door and go. That's all you want when you're in those early days.

BB: How do you deal with the toddler years?

HH: I think you need to work on yourself. Your toddler will do what they need to do and not necessarily what you say. That's just a truth. So you need to work on yourself. If you're patient, then they will be patient. If you're impatient, then they will be impatient. If you speak gently, they will be gentle. You set the mood. And you really have to decide what kind of person you want to be. Whatever you want them to be you have to start becoming.

ROCKIN' LIST MOM: SHARON OSBOURNE

When you're the wife of rocker Ozzy Osbourne and it's the day before Father's Day, it's up to you to think of something special. "We'll just pamper Ozzy all day long and give him his favorite foods," Sharon Osbourne tells Black Book.

Uh, we hate to ask: What are Ozzy's favorite foods? Bat heads à la mode? "No, he just loves my strawberry cake," Sharon, mother of three, confides.

We asked the mom of famous Kelly, Aimee, and Jack Osbourne for a few parenting tips, and she told us: "First of all, you shouldn't have a child unless you love the thought of being a parent and a good parent. It's all about unconditional love," she says.

"Your child must know that he or she is always safe," Sharon says. "Your child also must know that your home is a place of love and they're always loved in the home. I think that's what gives every child a good foundation to go out in the world, because they've grown up knowing that their parents love them. There is no end to the growth from there," Sharon says.

CHAPTER 7

Welcome to Sippy Cup Land (for New Moms)

Listening to my kids and encouraging them. That means more to me than any extravagant party or backyard full of snow.
—Tori Spelling

Gene Simmons's Rules of Parenting
1. Respect me.
2. Do as I say.
3. See first two.

DROP THE POUNDS BY SITTING DOWN

The last thing you have when you just had a baby is TIME. It is a thief, and you'll soon find out that there is never enough of it. However, you must take a seat if you want to drop weight. Researchers at the University of Toronto fed two groups a meal with the same number of calories; the first had lunch at a table (complete with linens); the second ate while standing at a kitchen counter (with baby on the hip no doubt). The results? The standers ate 75 percent more at their next meal.

So, new mommies, take a few moments for yourself and to teach your children early to respect their bodies by taking the time to eat your food in a civilized manner.

DO YOU WANT TO NUDDLE?

Celebrity moms like Angie Harmon have found a great way to nest with their newborns. Laying on the couch with your little one on your chest can be a taste of heaven, but you haven't experienced anything until you've done it with the amazingly comfortable robelike blanket called the Nuddle. Mom-prenure and creator Jenn Feldman has been featured on *Oprah* for her interior decorating skills. The new wife and mother says the extra-long cozy soft Nuddle, which is Cuddle + Nap = Nuddle, has slats for your arms to hold the remote or baby easily and an outer pocket for feet or to hold a pacifier, bottle, and snacks for your tiny tyke. The Nuddle is fifty-five inches wide and seventy-one inches long and is made out of ultra-plush microfiber. It goes for $110 at Nuddle blanket .com.

ANTI-BELLY-BLOATING DRINK

One thing you'll be hard-pressed to find on any Red Carpet is a bloated belly, even if you had a baby less than three months ago. It's true that celebrities seem to be able to make the bulging and extended bellies disappear. While skeptics claim it must to be immediate surgical tummy tucks after birth, we have our doubts it happens quite as often as reported. Here is a trick we learned from some of the best bodies on the beaches in southern California, and it can help new moms wanting to unload those unwanted pounds in the stomach region:

Into a large glass of cold water, place a few slivers of ginger, cucumber, and lemon, and a few sprigs of spearmint leaves. Drink eight glasses of this homemade concoction throughout the day to aid in eliminating belly bloat.

BB EXPERT: CATHERINE McCORD

"Did you know that babies love avocados? They're so nutritious and packed with vitamins. They're also really yummy," says Catherine McCord, who reminds us: "You don't know what your child will like until you try it."

The LA-based former model and culinary school grad has started a fabulous Web site we adore called Weelicious.com, which offers the best recipes for ultra-healthy baby and toddler food that is so yummy the adults in the family will be stealing the leftovers. Chicken salad with wild rice and grapes, anyone?

McCord tells her story: "I started modeling and traveling the world at a very young age, tasting and being turned on to foods that were exciting and exotic to my Kentucky-bred palate. When I was living in Paris, Milan, and New York and traveling to places like Tokyo, Morocco, and Sydney, I became obsessed with learning about local cuisine.

"Later I went to culinary school, then worked in a few restaurants trying to learn more tricks of the trade," she says. "Whenever people ask me what type of cuisine I like to cook the best, I say 'What's fresh?' The most important part of food is the ingredients you start with. I like simple food that speaks for itself."

McCord has an adorable toddler son named Kenya whom she exposes to seasonal, organic foods that are as pure as possible. "I want him to know that food shouldn't have to be pumped with sugar, salt, and preservatives to be delicious," says McCord. "Kenya only knows what I feed him. If I gave him McDonald's, he'd love it, but if I give him pesto chicken, that's what he'll crave."

BB: How did you start Weelicious.com?

CM: I started it off by having a child. I also went to culinary school and I wanted to cook for him. When you're a mom, you have two things: the baby and your computer, and that's it. For six months a lot of your outside world is that computer, and I wanted to get all the knowledge together that's necessary. Kids can be allergic to gluten, nuts, and dairy. It's very confusing and scary. You have this little baby and don't know what to give him. Meanwhile, we want our children to eat organic and we want to go to farmers' markets. We're not the Kraft mac-and-cheese generation.

BB: How do you introduce new healthy foods to your child?

CM: It's so much fun to turn your child on to new things. People said he'll never like beets, and he loved them. I'm the anti–Jessica Seinfeld. There has been this surge of cookbooks that say let's sneak food into our children's diets. Why are we sneaking? Let them eat these amazing fruits and vegetables from day one. Let them decide what they like. Why are we tricking our kids?

BB: What did your son eat that shocked you?

CM: Brussels sprouts and beets. We were taught to hate those foods. We were taught, "Don't make me eat broccoli." Instead of giving him a bag of Cheerios in the stroller, I give him bite-sized beets as a snack. They feel good on his gums and they're sweet. He loves them and they're delicious. Don't pick really red ones, though, because they get all over your baby and everything else.

BB: What do you avoid giving your child?

CM: I try to avoid sugar and processed foods. We have the highest child obesity rates in the world. I'm trying to show you can buy fresh organic food and it can be the same price as going out and buying food that's laden with sugar and salt and ingredients you can't pronounce. I take finances into consideration with all my recipes. It needs to be easy, fresh, and fast. And everything is good . . . I eat whole-wheat cinnamon banana pancakes, and they are great for the whole family. Again, I don't put sugar or salt in my recipes. I'm trying to keep him away from them for the first eighteen months. He has had bites of cake. I'm trying to train his palate not to crave sugar and turn him on to other things.

BB: If you have a picky child, what do you do?

CM: It's hard because it gets to be so frustrating. Most kids love my turkey meatloaf bites. Try foods the child can hold for himself or herself and foods that have good flavor but are packed with vegetables. My meatloaf bites aren't just ground turkey but also veggies and cheese, which adds flavor. Kids like what they can hold themselves.

BB: Are your Wee Nuggets like chicken nuggets?

CM: Yes, but they're baked and not overly oily. No goopy sauces. You could use ketchup as a dip, or you could take puréed tomatoes and make your own dip. Mustard is good, too. These Wee Nuggets are so quick. They take eight minutes to make, start to finish.

BB: What should moms always keep in the fridge and pantry?

CM: Pesto is great to always have on hand. It's olive oil and herbs, and you can put it on pasta or fish. It's so delicious, and you know it's not bad for you. The one thing I always have in the house is gallon sizes of purées I make out of fruits. If you have a baby with a sweet tooth, it's nice to have a homemade apricot purée to put on top of yogurt or use it to make curried chicken with the apricot purée. I add some raisins to the apricot purée, too. You can also put it into the meatloaf bites if you like.

BB: What do you do for snacks?

CM: You want things that aren't going to be all over the stroller, the car, and on your child. I'll take healthy crackers with nine grains or unsalted pretzels or raisins or dehydrated strawberries. My son loves those snacks, and he will always eat dehydrated fruits. Look for a company called Crispy Green—this company makes dehydrated bananas, apples, and pears. They're like chips but made out of fruit. I also have a dehydrator in my kitchen. I dehydrate sweet potatoes, bananas, and watermelon for him. They last for weeks, and they're great for teething babies. It's like jerky. It takes a long time for babies to break them down and it feels good on their gums. Rice cakes are also good to have on hand. I buy the ones with no sodium. There is another cracker my son Kenya loves called Finn Crisps. They're multigrain crisp crackers that are incredibly delicious. I went to a detox spa years ago and they gave us these crackers. Very healthy and delicious.

STAR BUYS

We admit it: There is no one who knows how to buy for the little bambinos like Hollywood starlets. Our friends at a great Web site called HealthyHollywood.com told us what some of the stars are buying for their newest costars:

- We love that Nicole Richie is all about going green when it comes to her baby daughter, Harlow. "I use Seventh Generation diapers, and we don't use baby wipes—we use cloth with water," says Richie. "We wash all of her clothes and my clothes in Seventh Generation organic wash."

- Tori Spelling knows all about balance with her son, Liam, two, and a newborn baby daughter. Her lifesaver is an Orbit stroller. "It's the best thing since sliced bread, because it's so functional," she explains. "It turns 360 degrees, it's portable, and as a car seat it's very secure."

- Jessica Alba says the best gift a new mom can buy herself is two extra pairs of hands. She says that her biggest present was some help. "I knew I would need a night nanny! Or someone to take care of the baby at night when the baby first comes home, to help you get acclimated," she says. The beautiful star of *The Fantastic Four* got a little more help from interior designer Kari Whitman, who helped her create a gorgeous pink, lavender, and white nursery that was also environmentally correct. "That's the way I live. Kari respects and shares my views on being as green as possible. I've been into anything eco-friendly or sustainable for a little while now, and I wanted to make this environment as nontoxic as possible. When I was doing research on furniture, I thought Nurseryworks was really cute. I told them I wanted formaldehyde-free wood and low-VOC [volatile organic compounds] paint, and they were like, 'That's our line.'" Alba says. Another perk is that the furniture grows up with your kids: The bed becomes a toddler trundle and the changing tables can be turned into a dresser.

Black Book Extra: Did you know that Alba also participated in hypno-birthing classes, which are all the rage in Hollywood? Newbie moms learn how to relax, which helps all your muscles to stay loose and not tighten up. A calm mama allows her body to naturally go into birth mode without stressing mom or baby.

- Holly Robinson Peete knows that kids on the go . . . always have to go! "The thing that I love the most is called a TravelJohn Junior. It's a portable potty," says the mom of twins Ryan and Rodney, ten, Robinson, five, and Roman, three. "It's rolled up into an O-shaped funnel. It's shaped so a girl can use it, too. TravelJohn Junior is the best-kept secret because every time you get ready to drive somewhere your kids have to pee."

- Elisabeth Hasselbeck of *The View* is balancing a tough job with being a mom to two tots under the age of four. What makes her life easier these days is her Ergo baby carrier and a Moby sling. "Both are lifesavers," says the mom of Grace, three, and six-month-old Taylor Thomas. "The Moby is so great because you just have to wrap the baby in it like a big Band-Aid. Then you can walk the baby around and he instantly falls asleep."

Kelly Preston isn't wiping tiny bottoms anymore because her son Jett is sixteen and gorgeous daughter Ella Bleu is eight. But she can still remember her new mom get-through-the-day tip: baby-wipe warmers. "The wipes are warm and don't really wake the baby up in the middle of the night," she says. "When they're all cozy and toasty-warm the baby wants a wipe that's the same. You take a warm baby and wipe them with a freezing cold wipe and they'll cry every time."

SISTERS AND MOTHERS

We love these twin sisters named Karla and Karen from Chicago who decided that they needed a little bit of help when their sons were little guys. "We lived within a mile of each other and were able to enjoy taking walks to the park with our children or being able to drop in on each other for a cup of coffee," the sisters say.

"Early in 2001, Karla and her family moved to Detroit. As a result of Karla's move," says her sister, Karen, "we found ourselves traveling back and forth between the two states much more than we ever imagined. During those trips Karla's son Alex kept throwing his sippy cup all over the car. After one particularly embarrassing flight Karla called me and said, "There has got to be something out there to stop this." They invented the No Throw cup. It fights tightly around and holds on to children's bottles and sippy cups. The No Throw's leash-style handle can be slipped over the seatbelts that are attached to your child's car seat, stroller, bike seat, high chair, baby-backpack, you name it. You can find the product at nothrow .com.

RED CARPET ARRIVAL

We don't know what will happen on the next episode of *Desperate Housewives* because we can't pen it ourselves. But there is one sort of drama that you, the new mom, can write from start to finish: your birth announcement.

Spread the word about your newborn's starring role in the world with 5starbaby.com birth announcements. They're not just boring little pieces of paper but movie poster mock-ups that cram details about the new arrival of Junior into one adorable ad.

Your baby's image is the feature presentation with marquee billing going to parents (producers) and doctor (director), relatives in the credits, effusive critical quotes, and more. Opt for an original title or take an existing one (*Little Miss Sunshine*, *Pretty in Pink*, *Sleeping Beauty*). That will get you boasting about your baby's, er, born identity—sorry, we couldn't resist.

SUNNY DAZE

Mothers like Nicole Kidman, Marcia Cross, and Naomi Watts have fair skin, light eyes, and light hair, and they are very conscientious about protecting themselves from the sun. However, add a newborn to the mix and you have celebrity mommies that can turn downright neurotic when it comes to raising their kids in the California sun almost twelve months of the year. That's why many moms go to such lengths to find the perfect sunscreen for their little one, and one of the most sought-after is LUCA Sunscreen.

Dr. Karl Gruber is a surgical pathologist in Charleston, South Carolina. He sees firsthand the damaging and often life-threatening effects of too much sun—and he's seeing this in younger and younger patients. Knowing that sun protection has to start early to be effective, he tried to apply sunscreen on his toddler son, Luca. But Luca was extremely allergic to every brand on the market. His allergies prompted Dr. Gruber and his wife, Georgia, to create LUCA Sunscreen, making it hypoallergenic, scent and oil free, water resistant, and with the highest UVA protection on the market. It also is the only sunscreen available in the United States that states its critical wavelength (383nm) on the bottle. Critical wavelength is how UVA is measured, and LUCA Sunscreen is better at blocking UVA radiation than other sunscreens sold in the United States, effectively shielding the skin for up to six hours from UV radiation, which has been linked to premature aging, skin cancer, and melanoma. LUCA is considered one of the best sunscreens available, and since it's hypoallergenic it's perfect for children and their parents.

TEETHING BLING

Denise Richards, Angela Bassett, Ming-Na Wen, and Tori Spelling are all mothers, but they're also fashion plates. That is why they all wear Teething Bling, the new, fashionable, cool, hip necklace that hangs on a black silk cord but also is a great baby-safe donut-shaped teething ring in one. It soothes sore gums and keeps baby occupied at the same time. You look good and keep your child quiet and happy at the same time. What could possibly be better than that? In fact, P. Diddy's former gal pal Kim Porter, mother of their twins, wears one with all of her designer outfits for her girls. The founders of Teething Bling tell us, "We started our company, Smart Mom, in 2002 as a way to promote pretty and practical ideas for real moms. The Teething Bling was inspired by babies who like to tug on our jewelry."

It's made from the same material as many teeth toys. And

now A-list grandmas, aunts, nannies, and even fathers are buying them as a way to bond with baby and have an interesting piece of jewelry at the same time. By the way, they're 100 percent lead-free, nontoxic and phthalate free. All pendants come with a breakaway clasp. You can buy them at smart momjewelry.com.

BB EXPERT: ABIGAIL SPENCER

Abigail Spencer is an actress on the rise. At twenty-six years old, she has been in the entertainment industry for nine years, starting at age seventeen on *All My Children*. "I worked with the most beautiful mother of two Susan Lucci and most amazing now mother of three Kelly Ripa! Talk about women who know their stuff," says Abigail, who is now pregnant. (Congrats from Kym and Cindy!)

"Susan and Kelly were huge inspirations to me on balancing motherhood and work, long before I was thinking about marriage and babies," she says. "Life just keeps happening and I just keep sitting back in awe! Another woman in my life who was balancing motherhood and career is my dear friend Kathie Lee Gifford. She was and is such a mentor and does it all with grace and ease, and she was a huge reason I got to meet the casting director *All My Children*."

Now living in Los Angeles and the star of several indie films and the series *Angela's Eyes*, Abby has guested on shows including *How I Met Your Mother*, *Bones*, *Ghost Whisperer*, *Moonlight*, *My Boys*, *CSI*, and *Gilmore Girls*.

"Since the beginning of my career, I've seen all these women making it work and living their lives and having their careers and families. They make it seem so natural," she says. "Now I'm getting the opportunity to go through the rite of passage. I'm twenty-five weeks pregnant as we speak and I've had such a glorious time thinking, dissecting, and experimenting with beauty in this new state of pregnancy, and trying to do it all with grace and ease, and the knowledge I probably won't do it with either.

"People keep stopping and asking me, 'What are you doing?' I love sharing my 'secrets,'" she says.

BB: As a successful actress, model, wife, and expectant mom, you have a busy life here in Los Angeles. Tell us a few of your secret beauty products that you use to keep your skin looking so flawless.

AS: The thing about me and beauty products is that I have been experimenting for almost ten years, and I really have found some things that work for me. It's all about trial and error, and trial and triumph! I started experimenting on my first job when I was seventeen years old after I'd signed on for two years at *All My Children* playing Becca Tyree. I moved to New York right out of high school from my little town of Gulf Breeze, Florida, and thought I was going to land on the sound stage and they were going to make me look beautiful every waking hour of the day, solve all my problems, and give me all the answers so I'd never, ever need to worry about beauty again. Uh, wrong! Actors have to work REALLY hard to figure it all out, and no matter how much it disgruntled me, no one was going to do the work for me. So this list is a conglomerate of the things that have worked best.

There are still a lot of products that I'm trying out and have had to change for my pregnancy, but if you are willing to put the effort in, it saves you a lot of time on the back end. I'm trying to figure these things out now, because I know I won't give a rat after the baby is born, or I'll care and won't have time, so here we go:

● Face Wash: Dial Soap

dialsoap.com

Out of all the things I've ever used, I keep coming back to Dial White Antibacterial Soap. I'll switch to something else, and it will just break me out or won't get my skin clean enough. Cheap as it is, it has worked, works in my pregnancy, and worked for years. (You have to use a good moisturizer when you use Dial. Don't go without it because it is somewhat drying, which is fine as long as you moisturize.)

● SK-II Products

sk2.com

This is a new product line for me and I love it! It's pricey, but I figure I'm saving so much with my Dial soap. You have to know where to spend and where to save. I discovered it after I briefly met Cate Blanchett. I was just floored with how flawless and lovely her skin is—it was the best I had ever seen. When I found out she used SK-II, I ran out and got it. In fact, I went to Saks and asked the sales gal if there was one thing from that line to buy, what would it be? She said Facial Treatment Essence. I also bought the Facial Treatment Masks and Facial Treatment Repair C in a gift set. It's all amazing. Apparently the secret ingredient comes from saki. Do not drink it. Seriously, don't.

● Arbonne

arbonne.com

Arbonne is an all-natural line of skin care that you can't buy at the store, only through a salesperson or the Web site. It's very reasonably priced and if you sign up you can get 35 percent off everything you buy. The two must-haves in my book are Nutrimin C Vitamin C Eye Cream and Nutrimin C Transforming Lift Serum. I truly feel I can't live without these products now. They have the best eye cream, and both of these products have been preventing that "mask effect" pregnancy brings.

Vanda Beauty Counselor Vitamin C Roll-On Ointment

vandabeautycounselor.com

This is a little-known small cosmetics company. The only way I know about it is because my mother sells it. But they have this Vitamin C Roll-On Ointment for your face—it's pure vitamin C. I've noticed such a difference with my skin. Every facialist or beauty expert I talk to says the only way to slow the aging process is vitamin C. This company has little tiny orange and clear bottles that are easy to apply, and full of the exact thing our skin will never get enough of. I love it! And it's less than ten dollars at health food stores or GNC.

Zapzyt

zapzyt.com

This is an inexpensive topical cream—about three dollars—for whiteheads and zits. You can find it at Wal-Mart and most drug stores, but only use it on the infected spot because it's very strong. If using during the day, apply with a Q-tip, let dry, then dab your concealer of choice over it. Nothing has gotten rid of my blemishes faster.

Jane Iredale Makeup

janeiredale.com

When I was working on the show *Angela's Eyes* the makeup artist and I went through a series of experiments. I was going to be working sixteen to eighteen hour days, act in almost every scene, and be in close-ups almost every second of the day, in every weather element. By the way, we were also shooting in HD—which I'm sure you've heard is not the kindest to the ladies. I'm not the type of person who should look like she's wearing makeup. I need something that accentuates, makes me look flawless, and makes it seem like I'm wearing nothing, so I don't start to look too, shall I say, "Lady Marmalade-ish." Nothing was working. Everything looked like too much on me, or if we didn't use enough, it didn't have enough coverage. Finally she found Jane Iredale Pressed Mineral Powder. I've never looked better on camera. It acts as a base, coverage, and powder and has SPF 20. It looked so good and so natural that I started using it in my everyday life. Since then every makeup artist I've worked with has switched to the Jane Iredale line and is using it on all their shoots. I use Golden Glow as my base and then Caramel to warm up the skin or create a bronzier look. It's the easiest, most fabulous makeup I've ever used, and that's saying a lot from someone who doesn't like makeup! Also get the Kabuki brush applicator. Using that brush in circular motions with the makeup helps with the "flawless coverage." I've been using my original product for two and half years and just now had to buy a new one. It's $48 per compact.

Shu Uemura Eyelash Curler

shuuemura.com

Just go to Sephora, buy it for $17, and use it. I've even stopped wearing mascara. I have a Twix commercial out right now, and the director didn't want me to wear mascara, but I wanted to look awake and like I had eyes. The Shu Uemura Eyelash Curler did the trick, and there was no mascara involved!

Prescriptives Flawless Skin Total Protection Concealer

prescriptives.com

This is the best concealer I've ever used. I use it under my eyes, on my blemishes, and anywhere else that needs highlighting. I have very thin skin under my eyes and it can look blueish, especially on camera. For some reason, this is the trick. Again, every makeup artist I've worked with has gone out and gotten it. I use the Level 2 Cool, but you have to match it to your skin tone and make sure that during pregnancy you use it on those masklike areas. It really evens them out.

SuperNutrition Prenatal and Postnatal Vitamins

supernutritionusa.com

Get them at Whole Foods. They are strong, so space them out during the day. These vitamins are the best because they have more of the folic acid, calcium, and everything than any other vitamin. My nails and hair have been growing like crazy, my hair is shiny, and all that good pregnancy stuff is happening. These vitamins have been my saving grace during pregnancy and have kept me moving. (In more ways than one—enough said.) What's on the outside starts on the inside, so all the beauty regimes and products are pointless without a good diet, exercise, lots of water, and a vitamin routine.

BB: What is your biggest feel good-secret of your pregnancy?

AS: My biggest feel-good secret is prayer, listening to my body, and not stressing. It even says it in the Bible: Do not worry! So, that's what I'm doing. I just keep trying to deal with all the twists, turns, and unknowns this phase of life offers without fear! I'm trying to see lots of movies, read lots of books, hang out with my friends, learn as much as I can, sleep a lot, eat a lot, and do whatever it is that my body is saying "DO NOW." It's working.

BB: What can't you live without during your pregnancy?

Alternative Apparel T-shirts
alternativeapparel.com/Collections/Women
The material, colors, and organic factor make them the most comfortable. There is such an array of styles, so I wore them from no belly, to some belly, to belly gone wild!

Lululemon Athletica
www.lululemon.com
Their Be Still Crop Pants in black are great for the expanding thighs during pregnancy and work in winter or summer, along with a top they make that has shelf bra and cups included so I don't have to wear so many layers and the girls stay up. Plus, it's long so that it's not riding up my bel-bel. A girlfriend told me that you should get Lululemon stuff at six months pregnant because that's what your body will go back to right after you have the baby—however you were at six months. I'm six months and one week, so I'm loading up! They finally figured out how to do activewear right.

Vince Sweaters
www.vince.com

My Vince long gray sweater was the best investment! (Plus, I got it on sale.) It's plush and has a safety pin attached instead of a button so I can pin it anywhere as my belly expands. One of my girlfriends who isn't pregnant and is very slim liked it so much she went and got one, too. It's an "any time of life" sweater. Really anything by Vince rocks, and their line that Pea in the Pod carries is really great, too.

Long, Thin, Vintage Necklaces and Scarves

I'm talking long—like you can wrap it around a couple times long. Find things that accent the ever-growing bosoms and hang around the belly area. These create a nice distraction and natural V-shape, and they look like a little decoration on your belly. I like to knot the necklaces right over my belly button. It creates this long V look against whatever you're wearing, which is naturally slimming. You can do this with scarves, but knot them higher and let the longer pieces go.

Flat Vintage Boots

Buy the ones that come up almost to the knee. It gives the calf a fuller look, which makes your impossible water-retaining legs look smaller. I wear my mom's vintage boots in a rustic brown; they have that great beat-up look. Make sure you put a good orthotic in them to protect your feet. Look around at second-hand and vintage stores to find great boots. I'm wearing a lot of dresses, so I just put the boots on and it automatically gives any dress a vintage feel. They're flat, so no falling—unless you're me and naturally clumsy. Speaking of dresses . . .

Vintage or Secondhand Tunics and Dresses

I've been having dress fever and just want to live in dresses! Since maternity and today's (and yesterday's for that matter) current dress styles aren't that different (tunics, A-lines, empire waist, baby-doll), I'm set and don't have to buy expensive maternity clothes. I've been checking out places like Buffalo Exchange and Crossroads or any secondhand place on Melrose, finding these great dresses and tunics that are way too big on me. And the best part is that they cost between ten and twenty dollars but are made out of really good fabrics. I take them to my local tailor and have them taken in for another ten to fifteen bucks. Now I have all these cute dresses that are made from great materials. They will fit me through the rest of my pregnancy because I feel like they were made for me. All for thirty-five bucks and under!

H&M and Zara

hm.com and *zara.com*

If you don't mind spending a little more or don't want to have to go to the tailor and refuse to go to a maternity shop, go to H&M and Zara. You can get a lot of great stuff for well under $100. So many of their tops and dresses are blousy and give room for the expanding pregnant body. I've gotten a lot of my tops and dresses at both of these places.

A Good Minimizing Bra

I'm sad to say I'm still on the hunt. The only one I have is one my sister-in-law gave me, and it's awesome. The first five months my boobs kept getting bigger, but nothing else did. I saw a friend I hadn't seen in a while and he thought I had gotten a boob job and wasn't pregnant! So, minimizers for my ladies. I want to keep things in balance.

BB: How have you kept in such good shape during your pregnancy? What are your plans to lose the baby weight after giving birth?

AS: Keeping in shape during pregnancy is a theoretical term at best for me. I'm trying to be healthy and balanced. I'm focusing on gaining the weight . . . gracefully. What I've always tried to do is be in great shape at every other time in my life, and before I got pregnant I was doing Pilates almost every day. So now that I am pregnant, I'm not stressing. . . . I've cut back significantly due to a very difficult first trimester because I was so sick! But now that I'm well into the second trimester, I'm occasionally hiking with three-pound hand weights and doing Pilates with a prenatal specialist. I do yoga at least once or twice a week. I'm also running around, hanging out with my girlfriends, and getting the nursery ready in our new home! That's the best exercise of all. Some of the best advice I was given is "your body is going to do what it's going to do, no matter what you do." We are all going to gain weight and be soft. And I've just been accepting. So I've tried to listen to my body at every point during the process, and I've got to tell you, it's been great. I'm so thankful for being pregnant. It's given me this "in-tune-ness" that I've never had with my body, and this makes me never want to ignore my body again!

BB: As a busy soon-to-be mom, how do you take care of yourself? Do you have any quick tips for beauty, diet, or exercise as a mom? Any stress relievers?

AS: A huge stress reliever for me is not having to take a long time to get ready. I have quite a full head of hair. Unruly hair. At times it's crazy, and curly, and living a separate, much more exciting life than I'm living. Something that I'll do from time to time is splurge and go in for a really great conditioning treatment and blow-out. Even if I haven't showered or I'm running around and haven't looked in the mirror for some strange reason, I feel that if my hair looks good, then I'm doing okay. I won't look SO scary. And because my hair is naturally on the dry side and I live in California where I'm pretty sure it's not going to rain that day, I usually don't touch my hair for at least a week after that blow-out. That has been my real saving grace. I just get up and shower and go. And I usually don't wear makeup, so I can get ready really fast, which makes me very happy. My husband says I'm just lazy—and he's right, but I like to call it "planned effective laziness." This gives me more time do things I'd rather be doing. And I just laugh when I show up somewhere on day seven and people tell me how "great my hair looks and it must've taken hours." It did take a lot of time . . . a week ago.

BB: What was the one item, food, clothing, or ritual that has helped you get through your pregnancy?

AS: The one thing that helped get me through my pregnancy was my husband. I truly could not, would not want, do not want, to do it without him. He has made it so much fun and such a ride. I highly recommend finding one of his caliber! He has come to every ultrasound, filmed every filmable moment, encouraged me in keeping my focus on the right things, and just made this experience so special. He has been my ritual. Being pregnant has given me this insatiable desire for life and a realization of how short it is. A wise man I know has said many times that "at the end of our lives, all we'll care about is how we loved." Nothing else.

Black Book Extra: Kym and Cindy are tearing up reading your words again. We think they're just beautiful.

Some other fun things that at times I felt I couldn't live without are:

- Whole Foods Sonoma chicken salad sandwiches on toasted whole-wheat bread with olive oil, pickles, cucumbers, tomatoes, and lettuce. It's a custom sandwich order, and it's so good! The chicken salad has grapes, pecans, and poppy seeds. DELISH!

- Sweet potato fries from The Counter in Santa Monica
  2901 Ocean Park Boulevard
  Santa Monica, California 90405
  310-399-8383
  Hands-down these are the best sweet potato fries in Los Angeles. I mean, if I didn't live here, I'd have to find a way to get them. Pregnancy favorite and lifesaver . . . oh, I might have to go get some today!

- Aroma Café
  4360 Tujunga Avenue
  Studio City, California 91604
  818-508-0677
  I eat there at least three times a week. I love the iced orange juice and blueberry bran muffin, warmed up with butter to go for breakfast, and for lunch the Wild Rice and Tofu Salad.

- Lemonade. I've just craved it! I've tried the lemonade at almost every place in the city.

BB: What is the best piece of advice you received about pregnancy and mothering?

AS: The best piece of advice was from my dear friend Katherine Wolf. We were doing a private Mommy and Me Pilates session with her then two-and-half-month-old son, James. I had been with her since the beginning of her pregnancy. In the middle of doing an extremely awkward and difficult Pilates move called Scrambled Egg, she stopped with her leg propped up in the air, turned to me, and through her faint panting said, "Abby, I highly recommend having children! It just fills you with this indescribable joy! It is THE best thing that has ever happened to me." Well, I almost burst into tears. I had been saying I wasn't ready and that I didn't want to have babies yet, but with her words something just leapt into my soul. At that moment, I was open to having a baby and a week later I found out that I was pregnant. So the best advice she gave me was to have children! I'm ever so grateful.

BB: What is the best piece of advice you can give to someone else about pregnancy and mothering?

AS: The best piece of advice I can give at this point is to make sure you're in a great marriage first. Don't have children to fix anything or distract. Make sure you really want to be a mother. It's an extension of your love for your husband. And the second piece of advice I'd give is: Do it. Don't think that you have to do this and not something else. Don't keep putting your life on the back burner for something else that will ultimately leave you lonely and feeling unfulfilled. Just live your life and everything will fall into place. Maybe it won't fall into place the way you thought it would, but it will fall into place the way that God intended.

BB: How do you feel about the pressure new moms seem to have nowadays about how they must look perfect, lose the baby weight, and get back to work five minutes after having a child?

AS: I don't personally feel any of those pressures per se. I'd like to lose the weight. I'd like to go back to work. I'd like, I'd like, I'd like . . . but, I don't want to miss anything and any moment of this experience with my husband, new babe, and family. So if the second the baby is born all I'm thinking about or feeling is all this pressure to lose weight or go back to work or have to look "perfect," then that's sad. Those thoughts really add no eternal value to my life or to the health and happiness of my baby and family. I think I'll just ignore that pressure. I just feel like things will happen naturally if I stay focused and get out of the way. We'll see what happens!

I think something funny and mildly encouraging is to remember that if a new mom looks perfect, goes back to work, or has lost all the weight immediately after the baby is born, people are always like, "What! I can't believe it!" They will think you got lipo or had some sort of tapeworm or cognitive gene that makes you inhuman. It's always some sort of shocked reaction . . . so I think it's encouraging to remember no one expects you to be ANY of those things. It's a surprise if you are . . . so just don't worry about it. We're always MUCH harder on ourselves. Don't surround yourself with people who have really weird expectations of you and are completely unsupportive downers. It might be time to take an inventory of who is in your life.

EYE SEE A HOT-LOOKING MAMA

We can't mention names (she would kill us), but a certain pop diva gave birth to twins recently and appears to be keen on keeping her looks intact. We know she dropped the weight in a nanosecond, but she also kept her face looking remarkably not so tired and stress free, thanks to her nanny and ordering a case of Elizabeth Grant Caviar Rejuvenating Eye Pads. A spokeswoman for the beauty product company says, "We sent them to her after she had the babies, and she loved them so much she had her press agent call and request more. She's got tired eyes and loves the way these soak right into her skin."

SEXY MAMA

The last thing you feel after having a baby is sexy . . . that is, unless your name is Gwyneth, J.Lo, or Halle. They were probably sexy delivering. Anyway, for the rest of us mere mortals it's not going to happen without some major intervention. Well, BB followers, you just got lucky.

The Pleasure Chest is one of the Hollywood hot spots (pun intended) for all your after the baby sensual and sexual needs. Admit it, it's been so long, your husband is wondering if you are thinking of joining a convent. Everyone from the Beverly Hills socialites, to starlets, to stay-at-home moms from the Valley head over to this 4,500-square-foot sex boutique to check out their wares and spice up their love life after baby.

The Pleasure Chest goes the extra mile, and this sex shop in the heart of Hollywood has a free personal shopper program that pairs customers with in-store experts to navigate the store's entire selection of goods . . . ur, goodies . . . from candles to videos to toys to dress-up. The store likens the service to having a personal shopper (not quite like Nordies or Neimans, we surmise) or even a personal trainer who helps acquaint you with a gym's fitness equipment. Store employees are there to help clients "meet their sexual goals." If all goes well, you could find yourself pregnant again, so navigate prudently.

ONE LIFE TO LIV

Liv Tyler says fighting off those demons in Middle Earth was easier than figuring everything out about parenting. The mother of little Milo admits that being a parent has surprised her—and even taught her a few things. "I've learned about compassion," Tyler says. "We all have these limits in life. I know for me I'm always wanting to give everyone advice, but everyone has to find their own way. I've learned through my son that we're all made up of different stuff, which is so great." Tyler says her job makes motherhood much easier on her than other mamas. "I had the great luxury of being able to take some time off, which is amazing. I feel so lucky that I was able to be there with my son."

Any advice on how to parent a son? Tyler muses, "My son's favorite thing is animals, which is so beautiful because we can enjoy that together. It's my job to teach him about the animals—and teach him everything. It's my job to teach him how to be a man. I want to teach him how to cook, how to grow a flower, how to find a movie he will love, how to mow the lawn. It's about taking this little man and teaching him everything under the sun."

CHAPTER 8

Billionaire Baby/ Budget Baby

I don't want to be my child's best friend. I want to be a mom. But I do want my child to come to me when there is a problem and a need to talk, so it's going to be about treading that line.

—Jessica Alba

In LaLa land, there is no expense that is too expensive when you're having a baby. In this chapter we wanted to fill you in on some of the most lavish baby buys, which we will counter with a few budget substitutes when warranted. Happy shopping!

Billionaire Baby: Halle Berry has everything she needs for that seven-pound, four-ounce girl she and boyfriend Gabriel Aubry welcomed last year. Though Halle's camp is keeping mum about the details, we can tell you that the couple reportedly has spent big bucks outfitting nurseries in their three homes. Our source says Halle went for "all whites and neutrals" while shopping at Petit Tresor in LA, where she scooped up everything from the sheets to the stuffed animals.

One rule: Everything had to be made with cotton that never had a mist of pesticide on it. "She's obsessed with organic," says our spy. Except for that $1,200 Mia Bossi leather diaper bag.

Billionaire Baby: New mama Jennifer Lopez is wasting no time spoiling her double bundles of joy. The twin tots will gurgle and coo beneath two crystal bunny chandeliers from Petit Tresor (a cool $1,250 each), and their barfy bibs will get tossed into $1,000 matching antique hampers.

Billionaire Baby: When you're Jessica Alba and ready to pop, there is only one thing to do: You must go shopping. We found that in her last days of being pregnant with little Honor Marie, the gorgeous *Fantastic Four* star ran over to Bel Bambini on Robertson Boulevard in Los Angeles, where she bought BornFree baby bottles and a Boppy pillow, which really does help make breast-feeding more comfortable for mama and baby. One shopper was quoted as saying, "She just seemed so relaxed."

Budget Baby: Want a great baby gift that doesn't cost a fortune but looks cool and unique? Whoopi Goldberg says that she loves giving Bloomers Baby Diaper Cakes. They're made out of very usable diapers but are oh-so-cute. We love the cake with the small pink roses for $68.95. There's also a cake with safari green daisies and a zebra design for $68. You can even go with the FAO Schwarz cake with a pink paisley design for $79.99. These "cakes" are also great centerpieces for a shower. "If you want to send a great gift, this is what you want," says Whoopi. "You can choose the size and do it for a lot of money or a little bit of money. They take care of you." The company also has amazing "birth day" presents for newborns. The boxed sets include baby T-shirts, hats, and diaper covers. Check it out at bloomersbaby.com.

Billionaire Baby: Angelina and Brad's kids have one with skulls and fire, Gwyneth Paltrow's little one is painted Granny Smith sparkle green and is covered in padded "apple" fabric, which reflects her name, and, as expected, Johnny Depp's children, Lilly-Rose and Jack, have pirates and skull bones all over theirs. We're referring to the custom-made specialty kids' wagons with wood frames that cost around $650. When celebrities have a bundle of joy you can bet they won't be pulling their tyke around in the old-fashioned, bumpy red wagons we all had as kids. Thanks to West Coast Wagons celebrity and lucky kids can have customized wagons. Suri Cruise prefers the High Boy style, which uses the Radio Flyer bottom pan, but everything else is hand-fabricated. The chassis allows for a higher wagon body and large aluminum tires for safety. They come with hand-painted flames or other designs and oak wood slats.

In contrast Ben Affleck and Jennifer Garner chose the Princess wagon version, powdercoated with the bottom pad, handle pad, and seat cover, with of course seatbelts included. You can also get a cargo rack for your 8 by 10 glossies and to hold your script. The design is hand-painted with jewels and sounds like a steal at $275 compared with the other styles. The best thing about these unique rides is why and how they started. The creator's two-year-old daughter was born with cerebral palsy and partially blind. When top neurosurgeons said she would be strapped down in a wheelchair her parents decided not to let that happen. Their little girl, whose name is Piper, grew to dislike her stroller; she could not get comfortable and toys would always fall off. While hospitalized after a seizure, her parents found the only way to get Piper to fall asleep was to pull her around in a wagon, and soon they realized the wagon was key. The family molded their wagon into the ultimate stroller, but better. By adding accessories the makers say you can store all your bags behind the wagon with the cargo carrier net, load the wagon with toys, attach a CD player, pull down the shade tent, and best of all, no matter where you go you, always have a happy baby. Visit westcoastwagons.com.

Billionaire Baby: It's good to be the little sweet pea of the Simpson clan. Ashlee Simpson is just one of a slew of celebs who took her tummy to LA's famed Petit Tresor. Pete Wentz's mama plunked down a cool grand on organic blankets, Adiri bottles, and the Huddy Buddy onesie. Who could resist a baby in a onesie that reads "I'm just like my Dad!"

Billionaire Baby: Hollywood gets a doctorate in pampering, and it's never too young to start with your little star. Kid spas and salons are popping up all over, and one of the best is Spa Di Dah in Los Angeles. It's the first spa that caters just to kids, and many celebs are bringing their tots there. They offer services for kids from birth on up. There's even the Mani and Pedi for baby eighteen months and younger(!) and this includes a safe and gentle cleansing nail trim, a massage of baby's hands and feet, and you may even choose to finish off with a baby nail polish—nontoxic, of course. There are airbrushed tattoos for baby (that are safe). They also have the Cupcake Manicure and Pedicure, complete with toppings, including sparkles, decals, and polka dot options. There are hair extensions for kids to add a little to any style. The clip-ins go in easily and come up easily. There is even a party-time up-do for little girls heading to their preschool red carpet event. We just love the Little Fishes treatment for after swimming to remove the chlorine. No word if little Violet and Suri have tried it yet.

Billionaire Baby/Budget Baby: Jennifer Lopez is known for going over the top in many aspects of her life, but now that she is a mother nothing but the "Very, Very Best" is good enough for the twins she and Mark Anthony call their own. Even when it comes to pacifiers, J.Lo goes all out. Her little ones are calmed with crystal-studded pacies costing a cool $120 each at aristabrat.com. Yikes! If you're more conservative with your money for the little rubber teething tools that go into baby's mouth and usually end up on the floor, then the sparkly munchkin bling version may be the one for you, at only $5.95 for two. Who cares if it gets lost or falls in the dirt—but get rid of it if it hits the earth! Check it out at Babyearth.com.

CHAPTER 9

Mommy Needs a Cocktail

A Time-Out to Hear from Our Leading Men

Her five-minute look is my favorite. She looks perfect unmade-up.

—Gavin Rossdale, rocker and hubby of our
favorite ultracool mother Gwen Stefani

I call them my Goddess trilogy.

—Woody Harrelson on his three daughters,
Deni, Zoe, and Makani

McDREAMY, THE PARENT

Just when you think he can't be more perfect, Patrick Dempsey also turns into a total doll—literally. He has a great doll based on his character in Disney's *Enchanted*. This fact thrills his young daughter Talula, who can have her Barbie hang out with her Daddy doll. "It was kind of surreal going home the other night. I'm resting on the couch and all of a sudden my little plastic doll face pops up behind my shoulder. My daughter was laughing and laughing," he says. "And then she grabs her Giselle doll and my daughter begins acting out the movie with her Giselle and her Daddy doll. My wife and I just watched and whispered to each other, 'She's really good!'" Dempsey also has twin sons, Darby and Sullivan. His best parenting tip is simple: "Guys need to take the kids from their wife. So what if they throw up on you. It's all just part of the process. You don't want to be that guy whose kids didn't throw up on him."

DAMON, THE DADDY

"Being a dad is just amazing," Matt Damon says. "These stages just go by and it's incredibly fast. There are all these little discoveries every single day. So much changes in that first year."

"She's walking now," he marvels when talking about his baby Isabelle. "She's only thirteen months old and she moves at warp speed.

"You just wake up one day and realize she has grown so much. You want that little baby back," says Damon, who got his wish because as we go to press with this book his wife is pregnant again.

Damon says that certain aspects of new fatherhood do confound him. "Right now, my daughter makes this sound like a crow. She screeches, 'Aw! Aw!' and then points at things. This morning she pointed at the ceiling. There's nothing there. She still did her crow sound and then she laughed.

"I don't know what's so funny about the ceiling, and I try to figure out what's in her head," he says. "Sometimes she will go 'Aw! Aw!' and I'll say, 'You want some milk?' And she laughs. That one I get."

He says that a recent co-family trip with the Afflecks for some surfing in Hawaii has provided some bonding between his daughter and little Violet Affleck. Damon expects that some-day the girls will be swapping lip gloss and borrowing each other's clothes.

"They're much closer than in age than Ben and I are," he says of their daughters. "If we do it right, they'll grow up to be best friends."

DADA DUTY IS COOL

Remember the old days when it was only the woman who was having the baby? The guys just showed up in the waiting room and then were reintroduced to the child when he or she learned to play soccer or baseball. Well, those days are over and Holly-wood hunks are leading the way with hands-on daddy dudes like Ben Affleck, Matt Damon, Danny Moder, and Gavin (Gwen's hubby). Case in point: Brad Pitt has been photographed all over Lela Land with the Storksak diaper baby bag hanging from his toned, taut guns. Of course, it is the coolest baby bag around, made of pebble cowhide leather, and is a cool messenger-style shape. It includes a padded changing mat to make things easy for Brad and insulated side pockets along with a cell phone holder. (He can make deals and get rid of poopy diapers from Shiloh at the same time!) With a hefty price tag of $198, there is a bonus after baby. This better and bigger bag is one that any hottie can use later as a gym bag or even to haul around a laptop!

McDADDY

Matthew McConaughey is no fool. The man is a first-time father to son Levi and is happy to ask for some sage parenting advice.

His frequent costar, and mom to Ryder, Kate Hudson is only happy to oblige, but first she wants to know what he thinks fatherhood will be like. What is his fantasy version of hunk father knows best?

"How will I change my life?" McConaughey, thirty-eight, poses. "Well, there are a lot of things in my life that I won't change. The child will have to come into my life and be a part of that life that I have with the child's mother.

"For instance, someone asked if I'll stop doing movie stunts because it's dangerous, and the answer is unequivably no. I don't want to be foolish, but I don't want to teach my child to be afraid of things," says McConaughey.

Hudson sits listening to him in a suite at the beachfront Casa Del Mar Hotel in Santa Monica, California. The muscular McConaughey, dressed in a form-fitting gray sweater and tight gray jeans, looks fondly at Hudson, who wears black jeans, a matching T-shirt, and a gray suit jacket.

"Well, what you will notice about fatherhood is it will change your sleeping patterns," says Hudson, twenty-eight, the mother of four-year-old Ryder Russell Robinson. "Matthew, you won't get to sleep anymore. I haven't slept in four years. But now I negotiate. I say, 'Ryder, please. I'll put on *Curious George.* Just let Mommy sleep for an hour.' But even when you're sleeping one eye is open and one ear is listening."

"But do you say things that your parents said to you?" asks a horrified McConaughey.

"You do say the worst thing," Hudson insists.

"Because I said so?" McConaughey interjects.

"I say it all the time," Hudson says with a giggle, and her handsome costar takes it out for a spin.

The ultra-hot McConaughey just had a child with his girlfriend, Brazilian model Camila Alves. "We're going to keep the trailers. We're going to travel," he says of his new life with the baby. "I do want my child to have some culture, too."

The sex symbol admits, "I do feel more adult and grown-up now. I don't feel any older. I actually feel a little younger these days. With Camila being pregnant, I think my days as a parent have begun. There are shifts in my thoughts of the future. It's not just about me. And that feels good. This just encompasses more quality in my life."

McConaughey says his life is more mature these days. "There is a shift in my thoughts for the future. It's not just a me, it's a we. It feels really, really good."

Overheard in a Beverly Hills Delivery Room: This forty-ish leading lady who just had a baby also had a major snit fit at the revamped Essex House Hotel in New York City. She was aghast that anyone would DARE come into the very public ladies room while Miss Star was breast-feeding her new daughter. The only problem was no one even knew she was in there, so it was only natural that they would also use the facilities. What is an upset star to do? She actually was heard calling her publicist and griping to him about her total lack of privacy . . . in a public place!

BACK IN BLACK

Our favorite comedian Jack Black is the proud father of two sons, who haven't seen his kid flick *Kung Fu Panda* just yet. "My son is only one. He doesn't have a concept of celebrity yet. Neither does my newborn baby boy.

"As for advice for new fathers, I'd say change the diapers. If you're the one who doesn't change the diapers, they sense it. They know later and think, 'You didn't change me.' You really have to involve yourself in all aspects. So I change the diapers. I get my hands dirty," he promises.

CHAPTER 10

The Busy Mom Cheat Sheet
Beauty/Diet/Life Tips for You, Mama

Younger is better if you've found the right man. Menopause and adolescence should never share the same household.
—**Barbara Harrison, on what age to have children**

You've got five minutes and you've got a baby—how can you get the most from your beauty moment? Here is the latest and greatest to look and feel your best:

- Want less pain per pluck? Clean up brows after you shower, when pores are open and hairs come out more easily.

- The added bonus of pale pink nail polish is that it shows chips less than dark hues do. To extend the life of your mani, apply a base coat, to which polish clings. Apply a glossy top coat nightly.

- A little navy shadow over your black eyeliner will make your tired eyes look much less red.

- For walking and losing weight, walking poles and Chung

Shi shoes can help you lose weight and eliminate cellulite. They're a different kind of sneakers that tone the hips, thighs, and calves. The curved bottom shoe works muscles in your lower body. They lessen cellulite as you walk around in them all day. They also improve posture, muscle tone, and core stability. The unique design, which replicates walking on an uneven surface, enhances calorie burning, increases blood circulation in the feet and legs, and strengthens the connective tissues of the ankle and knee joints. Furthermore, a gentle finger pressure provided by a rocker bar inside the shoe alternately relaxes and contracts the muscles in the lower body, leading to an improvement of muscular strength and endurance. They go for $250: call 1-888-FITFOOT or go to footsolutions.com.

Try a Walkvest, a vest with little mini-weights built in it to increase your load and help you burn more calories and lose weight faster as you walk. It goes for about $80; walkvest.com.

Use baby teething rings (freeze them) to reduce swelling of puffy eyes.

We have been hearing from all our Bev Hills girlfriends about a new and inexpensive product available at local drug stores in the Valley. Forget the $150 Crème de la Mer and $220 creams from Japan. There is a new, affordable antiaging product from Britain called No 7 Restore & Renew Beauty Serum. It's touted as the UK's bestselling antiaging serum and is developed by Boots skincare (which is available at Target). It boosts collagen levels, protects against further damage, and claims to visibly reduce the signs of aging in just four weeks. The best part is that you can forget about going to high-end department stores and purchasing the commercial lines. It's available at Longs, CVS, and several other stores nationwide.

- Extra virgin olive oil under the eyes will reduce fine lines.

- Use Jell-O for kids (and you) at the beach or pool as a treatment for sunburn. It's a fun and tasty way to keep your kids' minds off the pain. The cool, mushy substance helps to soothe a bright red burn from being in the sun all day. Green might be a better choice than red, as red could scare the kids instead of make them feel better about their already red skin. P.S.: It feels great.

- Look great and flush toxins from the body after having a baby by eating seaweed. It is no accident that the longest-lived people on earth are the Japanese, who make seaweed an important part of their diet. Studies show that it binds toxins in the body and flushes them from the system. Scientists have even found that it helps prevent breast, endometrial, and ovarian cancers. Try nori (used to wrap sushi), dulse, and kelp, available from health food stores—add to soups, salads, and rice dishes.

- Keep looking good all through your pregnancy by looking your best with cherry juice. Courteney Cox and Kate Bosworth swear by CherryPharm, an all-natural cherry juice filled with antioxidants. Dermatologists say the concentrated tart drink improves the skin's texture and helps reduce inflammation and age spots.

- Tulsi Tea, or Holy Basil tea, is know as the queen of herbs in Ayurvedic medicine. Tarcy Martyn, a fab skin care guru for stars like Madonna, swears that by sipping this tea you will reduce inflammation—a good idea after having a baby. It costs $4.99 at Whole Foods.

Your nails are a wreck, you haven't had time to sleep, shower, or brush your hair, let alone go out in public and set an appointment for a manicure at the salon all your (perfect) girlfriends visit. Have no fear, the Black Book girls are here. Rub a little clear lip gloss over your unpolished nail bed. This little trick will give your nails an instant healthy shine and make your hands look well-groomed. A bonus: The oils in the lip gloss will moisturize your cuticles a bit and even promote nail growth to boot!

Okay, you had the baby and expected to lose the weight right after the birth . . . WRONG. So here's a quick and easy trick to make your face look a little slimmer while you're in the process of losing the extra pounds. Eyebrow experts to the stars tell me they have their celebrity clients wear a thicker brow right after having a baby because it makes the eye area appear larger and the face then looks thinner. Every little trick helps, and you don't have time to pluck or wax them anyway!

One of the last things to lose after having a baby is back fat. It's like your hormones want to hang on to it no matter how much weight you lift or lose. Well, we can outsmart a little back fat. . . . According to celebrity stylists, invest in a slim cami to wear underneath shirts that button. It's a slimming look and doesn't cling to back fat. Look for thin material or silks.

The last thing you need after having a baby is extra fabric in the hip area. That's why when we checked with the top Beverly Hills seamstress in town about what the skinny post-pregnant girls do, she told us, "Oh darlings, they send all their pants, jeans, and trousers to us and have us cut out the pockets. It instantly gives you a slimmer hip."

Black Book Extra: You don't need a tailor or an expensive alterations person—just grab a pair of scissors and cut.

- Have you noticed how right after having a baby many celebrities, like Jennifer Garner, Katie Holmes, and Sarah Jessica Parker, go darker in their hair color? They said in interviews with us that they just want to be more "natural"—well, natural, schmatural. Hairdressers to the stars tell us that they encourage their clients to go darker because it creates shading and shadows around the face, which make them look slimmer!

CHAPTER 11

Essay from Kym
About Motherhood

From my late teens until I was about thirty years old I would tell people, "I'm not going to have any children." I was a career woman and wanted to conquer the world. Well, that was a lie. Just a way of protecting myself from the haunting doubts and fears that maybe I wouldn't be able to get pregnant, find Mr. Right, or be one of those "superwomen" who could balance it all. Interesting how powerful words and thoughts are . . . sometimes what you say or fear can become a self-fulfilling prophecy.

Starting at a young age I had a tremendous drive to become a TV reporter, and I focused on that fully until achieving it. I then interviewed an actor named Jerry Douglas, who portrays John Abbot on *The Young and the Restless*, and a year later we were married. I moved from a small town in upstate Michigan to Los Angeles, California. I was going to take LA by storm—or so I thought. It seems that Hollywood wasn't desperately waiting for a small-town reporter from Marquette, Michigan. So I pounded the pavement, becoming a tour guide at NBC Studios, taking odd reporting jobs, and doing infomercials and commercials for years till I finally landed a gig on E! Entertainment Network. A show on the family channel called *Home and*

Family shortly followed. Note the name of the show . . . because at that exact point in time, I had been married for more than ten years and was desperately trying to have a child.

My husband, who is more than twenty years older than me, had a vasectomy. We were told we needed to get it reversed and I had to then be put on fertility drugs so they could pinpoint my ovulation cycle to increase our chances. We did the surgery, the healing took months, then scare tissue had built up because of the length of time he had had the vasectomy. Our dream to have a child seemed to move further away from becoming a reality.

Be careful what you say. Words are powerful. Be careful what you fear; you can attract that very thing.

The years dragged on while all our friends and family got pregnant, had baby showers, and bore beautiful, healthy children, and it all seemed so effortless for them. And then there was me.

I threw myself into my career and more doors started to open. I was on *E! Weekly* and *Home and Family* was getting great ratings. I had become a daily TV family member, plus I was doing a syndicated radio show with Jim Brickman and had a few infomercials running. Also, I began doing pieces for our local number-one-rated morning show *Good Day LA*. I was the career woman I had always hoped I would be, but the problem was it didn't matter because all I wanted was a child. The gnawing in the pit of my stomach never went away . . . the job, acclaim, and money could never fill up the desire for a baby in my heart.

We took more desperate measures as I started to approach my mid-thirties. Three pricey failed IVF procedures followed, and then a Beverly Hills urologist suggested a $100 procedure of removing the sperm directly from my husband's epidermis. We would then race the sperm to my fertility clinic down the street and have the doctor insert it immediately into my uterus.

They could not use anesthesia on my husband for the procedure because it could compromise the fresh specimen. They used a very large needle and it was done in the office. Jerry, bless his heart, did this for more than a year. Month after month we would try and wait anxiously with our hearts in our laps. Then we would take the pregnancy test only to learn once again that it didn't work.

I would be devastated, cry for days, and go into a deep depression, all the while smiling and posing daily for the camera as if all was perfect in my world. It would take me another month to get over my disappointment and depression, then Jerry would pep talk me up again and we would give it another try. It seemed endless as we continued for seven more months. I could barely stand the cyclical roller-coaster we had gotten ourselves on, but I would not get off. The hospital, medical, and prescription bills mounted. Insurance covered none of it, but it was the emotional toll that was the true price we were paying.

I wanted a child more than anything in this world.

Finally, Jerry went in for another attempt at removal and the doctor informed him this would have to be the last one. His scar tissue had built up and he could no longer remove the sperm this way without potential damage to the body, so it would be our LAST TRY. Jerry decided he didn't want to add to my stress and didn't tell me the news. The weeks passed and I was too afraid to take a pregnancy test. After six weeks, Jerry insisted we go to a local drug store and pick up the five-dollar test. We went home and I waited a few hours to take the test. I didn't want to know for sure that I wasn't pregnant.

If I didn't take the test, I was still able to hold on to a glimmer of hope.

Finally, I did the test and handed it to my husband because I wasn't able to read it. Turning my back to him, I walked to the door of our Brentwood kitchen and stared out into the night, bracing myself for certain disappointment. Jerry read it and slowly walked up to me as the sad tears rolled down my face, Softly he whispered, "It worked, we're pregnant. And honey, it was our final chance!"

I fell into his arms, and from the depths of my soul I was crying tears of joy and gratefulness. After five and a half years of prayer, endless tears, struggle, and disappointments, it was a miracle. We were going to have a BABY!

I was on *Home and Family* and I was having a family of my own. How perfect it all seemed.

I had a flawless seven months of pregnancy where I was like a machine. Stopping my daily exercise workouts, only light walking for me in case it put to much strain on the baby, and I never had a sip of coffee or alcohol. I would not even eat a chocolate chip cookie because the caffeine in the chips might affect my child. I was on a mission to have the healthiest baby ever.

I gained forty pounds and had swollen feet and a protruding belly button that was always sore, but I was ecstatic every day.

One of the stars of *The Young and the Restless*, an actress named Tracey Bregman, threw me a gorgeous baby shower at the Beverly Hills Tennis Club. It was exquisite—a beautiful sunlit large-windowed room off the courts with champagne, salads, and a customized baby blue cake.

I had my hair and makeup done and I was feeling beautiful as I waltzed into a balloon-filled room where all my friends and family were waiting to celebrate. I thought, "This is all just picture perfect."

That evening as I returned home, I felt a little weird. The baby boy who had not stopped kicking, punching, and rotating around in my tummy since three months old had instantly become motionless. Not one movement. I was feeling sick and deathly tired. Jerry assured me this was normal, and we both chalked it up to an exciting day of celebrating and getting down to the wire of the pregnancy. I took to bed and then it started . . . the vomiting, the diarrhea, dry heaves. It was unbearable. I could not stand up or leave the toilet bowl. I was sweating and had a high fever. Green and pasty, I had a headache that was pounding. I thought, "How could this be happening? I didn't do anything wrong. I'm so far along. I never touched the champagne or the wine. I only had that one little piece of cheese from the cheese tower that was up against the window and a small salad."

Then as quickly as it had hit me, the sickness left. I felt fine, the fever lessened, I wasn't sick to my stomach anymore, and we both told ourselves it was probably a bad case of food poisoning mixed with nerves.

But the baby was still not moving. I mean, nothing; he was completely still.

I went to bed exhausted and at 4 a.m. woke up in a pool of water. I didn't realize that my water had broken and I was about to give birth. The contractions started and we barely made the call to the doctor and the short trip to Cedars-Sinai Hospital before I gave birth within twenty minutes to a three-pound boy who was almost seven weeks premature.

It really helped having an actor as a husband because when Hunter was born, he was totally blue and was not breathing. My husband strategically stood in front of the doctor, who was holding the baby in urgent mode trying to suction his lungs. I didn't know any of this was going on because of the drugs and the rapid pace it was all happening at. Jerry smiled and laughed, telling me how beautiful and blond our newborn son was, never taking his eyes off me, explaining calmly that the baby had a lot of mucus that they were easily suctioning out so he could breathe better. The whole time he was blocking my view of the totally blue child whose lungs were not yet developed. But I knew something wasn't right because I never heard a cry. The doctor never spanked him and I kept saying, "Why isn't my baby crying?"

He wasn't even breathing, let alone crying. As the doctor rushed out of the delivery room with the baby, he alerted the staff that they needed a specialist and immediately raced Hunter to the NICU. Our precious baby that we had cried, begged, prayed for, and dreamed of for so long was slipping away from us and no one knew why.

The specialist, who coincidentally had been on the set of *The Young and the Restless* just days before acting as a medical consultant for the show, recognized my husband and moved into emergency gear. He told us later that he didn't know what was wrong with our little boy but was faced with the immediate decision of choosing Antibiotic A or Antibiotic B to put intravenously into this sickly newborn that he was rapidly losing. He picked Antibiotic A and with help from a ventilator our baby began breathing. However, we were far from being out of the woods. Still no one knew what was wrong. Hunter was placed in an incubator and received more than three blood transfusions in five days. His weight plummeted to less than two pounds. The worst day of my life was having to leave the hospital not knowing what was wrong with my son, stepping into our new SUV baby-proofed van with the empty car seat in the back and the ice pack in my underwear with no baby in my arms.

Was this all just a bad dream? Was I ever really pregnant? How do you go through such a traumatizing event and walk out of the hospital childless? *How? How?*

We practically moved in to the hospital, but we couldn't touch or hold our baby; his immune system was so fragile. I would order myself not to cry; I needed to be strong for my little boy, who was literally fighting for his life, but the moment I walked through the glass doors in the NICU incubation room, the tears flowed, my body sobbed, and my heart broke. Jerry and I would sit for hours on end with just our fingers allowed in the incubator, singing and talking to him, looking and praying through the glass, begging God to just let him live.

A few days later, the Food and Drug Administration people came to our home asking me if I could go into detail with them about everything I ate the day before my delivery. They had narrowed it down to the one small cube of cheese from the Beverly Hills Tennis Club. They had pieced it together and tracked it to the cheese tower that had been placed right next to the window—the hot sun penetrating it for hours had "turned" the cheese and it had contracted the deadly strain of listeria. When I ate the small cube of infected cheese, I introduced listeria into my body. I was able to throw it off after a short bout of illness, but I had unknowingly passed the potentially fatal illness onto my unborn child in gestation. I remembered hearing on the news about a fatal listeria outbreak that came from cheese. A large group of Latino adults had been hospitalized and then died after contracting the disease. How could my little two-pound newborn possibly survive while grown men and women had died of the same thing?

Now that the hospital knew what was wrong, they could treat it more aggressively. Looking back, that doctor in the emergency room, the specialist who had been a consultant on Jerry's show just days before, had made the critical decision between Antibiotic A and Antibiotic B. He didn't know it then, but Antibiotic B did not have the power to kill the fatal bacteria in my son's body. The doctor had a fifty-fifty chance of being right. He had chosen Antibiotic A and it killed the listeria strain.

For two and a half long weeks it was touch and go with Hunter, and I walked around in a catatonic state, smiling at the people in the hospital, talking politely to friends and well-wishers on the phone, and even agreeing to a televised call in to update the many *Home and Family* viewers who were concerned about Hunter's condition. I don't remember any of it. I was in a coma of sadness and fear, and all I did was cry and pray.

They told us if Hunter would take to the soy formula bottle, which I could now hold and give to him, that would be the test to see if he could sustain and fight off any potential infection or bacteria. Slowly but steadily I sat down into the rocking chair the nurses in NICU provided. Lifting him gingerly with all the intravenous tubes and needles attached to his little body and head into my lap, it was the first time I held my son, who was now more than two weeks old.

It was the most overwhelmingly beautiful feeling I had ever had in my life—more precious than anything in the world. He was finally in his mother's arms. Still and quiet, he looked up at me as I gently tipped the tiny preemie bottle to his lips. First he turned away, unsure of his sucking instincts, which were not kicking in. I got nervous and started shaking.

"Ohhh please, please drink from this bottle," I prayed. Then as if God's own hand reached down and turned his tiny head, his lips took to the bottle and he never stopped drinking. I'm not sure which flowed more steadily, the milk from the bottle or the tears streaming down my eyes.

We had won the first battle, but the doctors were quick to point out the war was not over. Being born almost seven weeks premature with a disease like listeria was a very precarious start to life. Hunter's immune system had been compromised and his lungs were not developed fully before birth. Having heavy medication and blood transfusions would most likely cause some damage. The doctors warned that he could be deaf from the drugs, his mobility skills might be delayed or even permanently affected because of the early traumatic birth, and they really didn't know how many other serious aliments he could develop down the road. The doctors told us we should not be too optimistic.

We didn't care and didn't even really hear the laundry list of impediments they were mentioning. Jerry and I were holding our newborn son, who was breathing on his own. He had taken his first formula and we could leave the hospital and bring him home, possibly within days.

The millions of viewers from *Home and Family* called,

e-mailed, and prayed for Hunter. We received letters from people of the Catholic faith who would go to Mass each day and light a candle for Hunter. There were Christian people who put him on twenty-four-hour prayers chains, Buddhist viewers who meditated for hours for Hunter's restored health, and Jewish people who were praying in synagogues and temple on Saturdays for our young premature son. All faiths, all ages, various ethnic groups, and just about everyone had rallied together for the little boy who was so wanted.

Our intimate friends and family called the prayer tower. They went to our church and had it mentioned from the pulpit; entire congregations lifted in prayer for him.

And Hunter slept, ate, grew, and flourished like no one expected him to. He never got sick with any infection or bacteria that could have been fatal if it happened in those first few months we were home from the hospital.

Hunter is ten years old now, and he is hardly ever sick and has never had an ear infection or any trouble with his ears. As a matter of fact, he hears so well that when his father and I are in our room at the end of the hallway whispering, he can hear it perfectly. We think his hearing is a little too good!

He goes to a school that excels in athletics, and he is the captain of his basketball and football teams. He plays soccer and is one of the fastest runners in his grade. His mobility skills are excellent, and most important, he has a tender heart.

The prayer and positive thoughts of millions of people are a powerful thing. I know for sure that love and kindness can change everything.

We truly believe that Hunter is a miracle—our miracle with God's help and divine blessing. We will never stop telling him that. We fully believe we had to go through this test of faith to appreciate the blessing of him. We know beyond a shadow of a doubt that it was God's hand that touched our child and made a broken premature newborn whole and strong.

We are humbled and will be forever grateful to all who were a part of our child's healing. Being pregnant with Hunter was one of happiest times of my life.

Happy pregnancy.

—Kym, Jerry, and Hunter

Our Favorite Story About Parenting
Indian Rite of Passage

Do you know the legend of the Cherokee Indian youth's rite of passage? His father takes him into the forest, blindfolds him, and leaves him alone. He is required to sit on a stump the whole night and not remove the blindfold until the rays of the morning sun shine through it. He cannot cry out for help to anyone. Once he survives the night, he is a man.

He cannot tell the other boys of this experience, because each lad must come into manhood on his own. The boy is naturally terrified because he can hear all kinds of scary noises. He figures wild animals are all around him and there could even be a human who might cause him harm.

Yet the boy didn't move and sat stoically, never removing his blindfold. It was the only way he could become a man! After a very scary night, the worst in his life, he felt the first rays of sunlight on his little face. He took his blindfold off and then smiled. He saw that his father had been sitting on the stump next to him and he had been there the entire night. He wouldn't allow one bit of harm to touch his precious little boy, who wasn't so much of a man that he didn't need his father's love and protection.

It wasn't just about being a man. It was about being a parent.

Wait, we're not done. We also love this story from Diane Keaton.

BB MOM TALE OF WOW

"There was a time in my life when I was younger and the days were just endless. Now it's nothing but events at my house," says screen legend Diane Keaton, mom to two adopted children, Dexter and Duke. "Oh my God, the other day, my twelve-year-old, Dexter, had an emergency with his pet rat, Baby O. I'm reading to my son Duke and about to go to sleep and I hear screaming coming from the bathroom. We both run into Dexter's room. Baby O the rat was drowning in the toilet like a reenactment of the movie *Ratatouille*. Yes, he was a drowned rat. Dexter said, 'Mom, I don't care what time it is, we have to take Baby O to the ER. We have to call an ambulance.' A friend of mine who was over had a better idea. We took my best hairdryer out and suddenly we were blow-drying Baby O like we were running a rat salon. We were drying out the baby."

AND BEFORE WE GO: MOMS MOVE MOUNTAINS

Here's how moms from the A-list and everywhere else can give back to help children around the world. Remember that no one wins unless everyone wins.

Below are three great charities to donate to when you get a chance. We love them because they help moms and kids.

Soles4Souls. Give your old shoes to kids in more than forty countries around the world.

GiveShoes.org

Nike Reuse-A-Shoe. Give old sneakers from kids and parents. Nike turns them into new basketball courts, tennis courts, and play surfaces for needy kids.

letmeplay.com/reuseashoe

Dress for Success. Help disadvantaged moms and women interviewing for jobs by donating your used but still good professional outfits and shoes.

DressforSuccess.org

If you bungle raising your children, I don't think whatever else you do well matters very much.
                    —Jacqueline Bouvier Kennedy Onassis

THANK YOU

Kym's Acknowledgments

First, I would like to thank the phenomenal woman who made this project possible: our editor and friend, Cherise Fisher at Penguin. She has helped to guide and direct us and she has seen the passion and potential of the Black Book series and franchise, and it has made all the difference. Thank you, Cherise, for being a champion for us. You gave the green light to *The Black Book of Hollywood Pregnancy Secrets* and then you got pregnant. Hey, maybe there is a connection. Blessings and congratulations on your own new chapter of life!

Elizabeth Keenan is publicist extraordinaire. Blonde, beautiful, and head cheerleader of the Black Book series, she has been with us from the start and holds so much credit for its successes. Liz, I adore you, you know that, and when can we go shopping in NYC?

What an honor to be able to say we have the legendary Jan Miller as our literary agent. She is the cream of the crop and her success is second to none in this business. Thank you for taking us into your literary family. We will always be your Black Book girls and there are so many more to come.

Nena, Nena, Nena Medonia. When we started with you, you were an assistant; now you are a power broker in your own right and you earned every bit of it. I think you are the BEST. Your faith leads you, and your intelligence and talent have moved you forward. The sky is the limit for you. So glad we have been on this ride with you.

To Jennifer Coles, my wonderful agent at AKA. Thank you for seeing the vision with me and for knowing that this is only the beginning for us.

Cindy Pearlman, my cowriter and friend, our pairing is better than George and Gracie, Abbott and Costello, Lucy and Ethel, Laverne and Shirley. You are my soul mate and we share so much more than writing—we share our hearts in our partnership and in our books. Cindy, you are full of beauty, grace, kindness, and tons of talent. Thanks for sharing it with me. XOXO.

To the other two children in my life, Avra Douglas and Jod Kaftan. I was thrown headfirst into stepparenting and didn't know how to swim, but we made it and I love and adore both of you. Thank you for teaching me lessons I could never have learned any other way.

How could I be a mom, stepmother, wife, daughter, writer, reporter, and correspondent without the help of my friends. I don't believe it takes a village; I believe it takes a strong family and selfless, giving friends who are always there for you. I have the best of the bunch:

John Livesay—thank you for the hours of encouragement and guidance, you bless me every day. Kristi Sindt, Robyn Dunn, Allison Gray Smith, Clay Adkins, Cynthia Pasquella, Matt Wright, Lisa Kridos, and Nicole Prentice, I could not do it without you.

My husband of twenty-five years (yay) Jerry Douglas. You have your priorities so straight. Faith, family, and then all the other stuff. Thanks for never putting acting, Hollywood, *The*

Young and the Restless, or anything before us! And as you always say, "A team that won't be beat can't be beat." So glad you're on my team.

Last, my precious mother and father, Barbara and John Bankier, who have been married over fifty years. You taught me that my faith in God had to be the first priority and all else would fall into place, because as Paul Johnson has on his office wall from the Bible: "What does it profit a man if he gains the whole world and loses his own soul?" You are my idols and my role models. It all started with you. Coming over from Scotland as penniless immigrants all those years ago on the *Queen Mary*, did you ever think?

Cindy's Acknowledgments

Thanks to amazing editor and champion Cherise Fisher at Penguin, who has guided the Black Books from the start. It is an honor and a joy to work with you. Thank you for taking a chance on us. Your encouragement is inspiring and insight is phenomenal. And on a personal note, congratulations! Love and best wishes!

Thanks to Elizabeth Keenan, one of the very best publicists in this business, hands down. You were instrumental in making the first and second books a success. Thank you for all of your hard work, savvy, and spirit. You're the best.

Thanks to the amazing Jan Miller for your guidance and belief in this project. Several years ago you started a journey with the Black Book that has been fantastic. Thank you for taking an idea and turning it into a book franchise. Your amazing insight and advice has made this project what it is today.

Nena Medonia. What would we do without you? You are the one who handles everything Black Book–related with such grace, charm, and diligence. You have guided us from the start with wonderful friendship and humor, too. Thank you for always being a phone call away and for being our biggest cheer-leader with this project. You're awesome.

Richard Abate, for your belief in me, amazing guidance over the years, and never-ending support of my dream projects. It is my honor, joy, and pleasure to work with you.

To Kym Douglas. I don't know what I enjoy more—writing these with you or laughing with you over all of the great things that happen to us along the way. Kym, you're a great cowriter and an even more amazing friend. I marvel at how you work so hard with such amazing faith, class, and, yes, fashion sense (come on, this is the Black Book). You and I are a great team with many more exciting things to come in the future.

Endless thanks to the other great editors in my life. Thanks to John Barron, Amanda Barrett, Miriam Di Nunzio, Avis Weathersbee, Darel Jevens, Laura Emerick, and Tom Connor at the *Chicago Sun-Times* for your many years of wonderful friend-ship and support. Thanks to amazing editor Gayden Wren at the *New York Times* syndicate.

To Joyce, Sally, and Vickie, three of the best friends a girl could be lucky enough to have in life.

Thanks to my brother and attorney, Gavin M. Pearlman, for looking out for my best interests and for your love. Love to Jill, Reid, Cade, and baby Wylie Jane. Thanks and love to Richard and Cheryl Pearlman, Jason, Kim, Craig, and Beth, plus Nathan and Max.

Thanks to my father, Paul Pearlman, for a lifetime of sup-port and love.

Get More
Celebrity Secrets

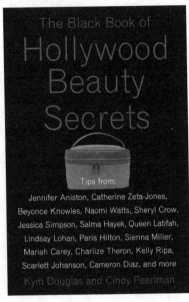

ISBN 978-0-452-28765-5

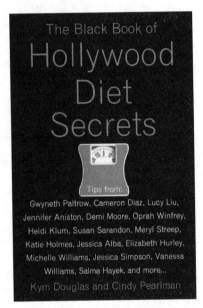

ISBN 978-0-452-28904-8

Available wherever books are sold.

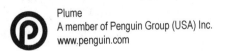

Plume
A member of Penguin Group (USA) Inc.
www.penguin.com